Mind Over Fat Matters

Mind Over Fat Matters

✦

Conquering Psychological Barriers to Weight Management

Lavinia Rodriguez, Ph.D.

iUniverse, Inc.
New York Bloomington

Mind Over Fat Matters

Conquering Psychological Barriers to Weight Management

iUniverse books may be ordered through booksellers or by contacting:

iUniverse
1663 Liberty Drive
Bloomington, IN 47403
www.iuniverse.com
1-800-Authors (1-800-288-4677)

ISBN: 978-1-4401-0228-8 (pbk)
ISBN: 978-1-4401-0229-5 (ebk)

Printed in the United States of America

iUniverse Rev. date 10/29/08

Dedication

For my father, Papi (1927–2001), who loved me unconditionally.

For my mother, Mami, whose many traits I am proud to have.

For my husband, Ed, the love of my life.

Acknowledgments

I want to thank my husband for believing in me even when I didn't believe in myself as a writer, for supporting me even when it meant he had to sacrifice something of his own, for providing humor at the precise moment that it was needed, and for making me feel loved at all times.

A special thanks goes to the many patients whom I treated throughout many years for trusting me and helping me to learn what does and doesn't work when it comes to successfully losing and maintaining a healthy weight.

Finally, I am grateful to Connie, my gifted editor and friend. We struggled together on this book and came out at the other end each stronger and wiser than when we started.

Introduction

For the last 30 years, Americans have been experiencing one of the most destructive epidemics of our time. There's no particular organism or person to pin it on and it's completely treatable, as well as, preventable. It is America's obsession with weight and dieting. It's reflected in the incessant messages Americans get that they're not thin enough and, therefore, not fully acceptable. Monthly articles in popular magazines show the latest in diets and promise success with weight, in particular, and with life, in general. Every year there's a new "Diet-of-all-Diets" diet. Scores of Americans will buy into it, despite having proved to themselves — year after year and diet after diet — that no miracle diet exists.

The latest "Diet-of-all-Diets" is the "High-Protein, Lo-Carb Diet." Forget about the fact that it's not a new diet (it was a fad diet when I was in high school, some 30 years ago). Actually, most new fad diets are not new at all. They're recycled. Why? Well, they made tons of money the first time, why not again? Obviously, the diet didn't work the first time or we wouldn't be on it again. Most of the folks on the diet are the same ones who were on it 30 years ago.

A friend recently visited me with her daughter in order to spend some time enjoying the outdoors. I prepared lots of healthy stuff for lunch. I made fresh, whole-grain bread, and served fruit, turkey, cheese, juices, and other appetizing tidbits. Oh, Oh. They can't eat *any* "carbs." They're on the "High (All) Protein Diet." They'll have just turkey and cheese (and a diet soda, of course). So we sit to eat...I, eating healthy grains, fruit, and protein; they, picking on slices of no-fiber, low nutritional value, fatty, cheese and meat. Okay, to each his own but, curiously, I'm the thinnest one.

Today, my landscaper was working hard on one of my many great ideas. I made sure there was good food to offer him during his break. "Oh, no, I don't do carbs. I only eat protein. I brought my cheese with me. I'll have a diet soda, though."

What is this? He certainly looks lean, but how healthy is his heart, I wonder. Come to think of it, I've never known him *not* to be on a diet. Oh, well, to each his own. It's harmless, right?

What Is This Book About?

If you…
…are overweight,
…are ready to give up unsuccessful weight-loss methods,
…want to become lean and fit,
…want it to last a lifetime,
…and want to enjoy the process,
…then you are in the right place at the right time.

What This Book Does Not Do

This book does not promise…
…to make you lose weight with no effort on your part,
…to make you look exactly the way you always wanted,
…to make you lose all the weight you wanted, or
…to make you happy.

What This Book Can Do

This book can…
…teach you what things have been keeping you from being successful with weight and fitness,
…teach you how to change such things,
…help you learn more about losing weight and getting fit than the majority of the people you know,
…help you be more successful with your weight and fitness than most Americans,
…be fun.

Part I

Building a Strong Foundation

Chapter 1

Friend or Foe: The Psychology

of Your Brain

"The brain is a terrible thing to waste." How true is this! The human brain is a complex and fascinating instrument, a great tool. Like any tool, to make the best use of it, you must know how to use it. If not used wisely and skillfully, it can be a detriment rather than an aid. In no other area does this ring as true as in trying to achieve a healthy and lean body.

Does this sound familiar? You want to lose weight and vow to stay away from sweets. Before long, sweets are all you can think about. With everyone else being able to eat sweets, you know exactly where the sweets are in the kitchen. The fantasy of being able to have sweets again is almost unbearable. In fact, sweets are remembered as the tastiest foods of all.

Is this fair? After all, you're trying to do a good thing. Why must your body resist the good intentions? You needn't be so hard on yourself. It's not you. You're not weak. It's just that the way we humans use our brains is a little out of whack.

Humans are not the only animals to show this seemingly strange behavior of resisting what they want or have vowed to do, nor does this happen with everything we vow to do. You may even be one of those few who usually does whatever they've set their minds to do. You may only seem to have

3

trouble following your intentions with dieting and exercise. It's still not your fault. You just don't know how to use your brain to your advantage.

Dogs and cats show the same tendencies (as do other animals). Does your pet get more excited about the food it's allowed to eat whenever it wants, or does it dance around more for its "treats?" If you have a normal pet, it gets more excited about the food that it likes but that is limited. We're no different from our pets.

I don't like spinach. I'm glad I don't like spinach because, if I liked spinach, I'd eat it all the time, and I don't like spinach (just a joke I heard somewhere). Anyway, I dislike spinach intensely. If they passed a law tomorrow outlawing the eating of spinach, I would have no trouble being a law-abiding citizen. However, I am a bread connoisseur. I have a reputation when it comes to liking bread. You can bet I would be an outlaw before long if bread were against the law.

"So what's so enlightening about that?" you might ask. Well, it's exactly what we do to ourselves when we diet. We set rules that prohibit the very foods we like and, often, try to make ourselves eat foods we don't like (just because they're lower in fat, calories, or are considered healthier).

It just happens that very few (I haven't met any) people consider vegetables their very favorite food and complain of craving them to the extent that they can lose control with eating them. The tastiest foods tend to have more fat and/or sugar. That's why brownies are so good. We have evolved to like fat. It has the most concentrated calories of any food substance, so you can get your daily requirement of calories in a smaller package. At one time, this was very useful. Food was hard to come by and we had to put a lot of effort into finding it before we could eat it. Better to hunt for the fattiest source. Our lives depended on it.

We're much luckier now. We can just sit in our car, drive to the supermarket, and pick up a nice little package of fat. The only problem is that our bodies are built to store fat efficiently and, since we don't have to work so hard to get food anymore, we get fat. That wouldn't be as much of a problem if we found it attractive as people did when only the rich could afford lots of food. If you were fat, we knew you had a lot of money and didn't have to work much — lucky you!

There is another problem with excess fat. It can cause a lot of health problems. This is its most serious problem but, in our culture, we're still thinking it's better to look "mahvelous" than to feel "mahvelous." I don't agree with this, mind you.

When we think of dieting or exercising, most of us think of something depriving and requiring a lot of effort. Who in their right mind would want to do something that's going to cause so much discomfort? Now you see how sane we've been to resist all those diets and exercise programs?

Children are lucky. Adults spend a lot of time studying what children like and consider fun. That's because if we can figure this out, we can get them to do what we want. The toy industry spends millions, if not billions, learning about what makes kids tick.

For some reason, once we become adults, we're just supposed to "do it!" DISCIPLINE. That's the keyword of adulthood. "BALONEY!" We still have the same brain we had as children. It still functions basically the same. The more fun, enjoyable, or positive we imagine something to be, the more likely that we will approach it or do it.

It's not difficult to see why we have so much trouble with dieting and exercise. We view them as things that we have to — must, should, ought to — do. It's "the best thing for us." Not only does this not sound like something fun or enjoyable, but also, if we don't do it, we have to feel GUILT. Yuck! Now it sounds like torture. Why would we ever expect ourselves to succeed under these conditions?

I hope you are convinced by now that the traditional "American Way" of dieting and exercise is not for you (nor for anyone). You may be all gung-ho and ready to learn to use that brain of yours the way it was intended. But first you need a foundation — some basics that will help things make more sense and make change easier.

Chapter 1 Tidbits

- The brain wants to do what it imagines to be enjoyable and resists what it thinks will be too much effort or discomfort.
- Most diets and exercise regimens are depriving and too uncomfortable, so people often have trouble following their intentions with diet and exercise.
- To achieve success with diet and exercise, we have to change our concept of how and why we should get fitter, and what we will do to achieve it.
- If it's not enjoyable, it's bound to fail — so why do it the same old way again?

My "Mind Over Fat Matters" Notes

What I want to remember:

What I want to do:

How this will enrich my life:

Chapter 2

Simple 1-2-3

The Basics of Successful Weight Loss

You wouldn't expect a child to read a book or write a letter without teaching him or her the basics — the ABCs and such. Learning is like building blocks. Everything you learn was built on a foundation of everything you have learned before. It is the same with fitness and weight loss. Without the right foundation you're not likely to succeed. Don't fret, though. The amount of information needed to learn to be successful with weight and exercise is very limited and simple.

The basics of successful weight loss are:

- Exercise

- Nutrition

- Eliminating dieting (any eating plan that severely restricts calories, fats, or particular foods).

What you have to know about each of these is easy and simple to follow. After learning these simple concepts, you will know more about nutrition, exercise, and dieting than most people.

Forget the word exercise. It's just a form of movement. It's movement that you want — movement that is easy, fun, and frequent enough to get the job done.

Why is movement important in losing fat? Because when you move, your metabolism increases. That means that it burns more calories in order to provide energy for whatever it is that you're doing. Calories in your body are stored as fat. You want to get rid of excess fat, right? So moving is a good thing — a very good thing.

If you burn fewer calories than you take in (eating), the extra calories are stored (fat). That would be a good thing if calories were money. Saving money is smart. Storing excess fat when you don't need it is not.

There are mainly two types of movement that you want to be concerned about. The first is the regular moving you do just going through your typical days. You get up in the morning at a particular time, have breakfast, maybe let the cats out, do a little gardening, have lunch…you get the picture. You might call this "lifestyle." Some people have a more active lifestyle than others (they move more from day to day).

My friend Delaney usually gets up no earlier than 11:00 a.m. She stays in her pajamas all day long unless she has to go out, and that's not often. She spends lots of hours in front of the computer (often late into the night). She eats her meals somewhere in between all this and goes to bed. Delaney is very overweight.

In contrast, my friend, Priscilla, gets up before 8:00 a.m. She goes down the stairs to get her coffee and attend to her cats. Depending on what day it is, she may clean house, swim in her pool, play tennis, or play golf. She eats her three meals during the day. My friend, Priscilla, has never been overweight.

Obviously, Priscilla has a more active lifestyle and, as a result, burns more fat. Delaney would be rich if calories were money. She has saved a lot during the years.

The second form of movement about which you need to be concerned is what is typically called "exercise." This is a regular activity that you consciously add to your lifestyle and that you sustain long enough to sufficiently increase your metabolism to efficiently burn fat. It could be a hobby, a sport, or an exercise program. It could be dancing, jogging, swimming, climbing stairs, walking, jumping up and down — the list is endless. If all you do is march while waving your arms, it qualifies as exercise.

Why is this form of movement important to losing fat? It just so happens that it has a nifty side effect. When you are doing this type of exercise, not only do you burn the fat required to perform the activity, but also your metabolism is increased for hours afterward. If you do this type of exercise regularly, you can conceivably increase your calorie burning on a daily basis. You'd be more like Priscilla and less like Delaney.

Let me clarify what I mean by sustained movement. It means moving at a pace that is not strenuous (able to talk while you're moving) for at least 20 minutes. It should be exerting enough to cause deep breathing. If you're out of breath, you're pushing too hard. If you're breathing like you normally do when you're not being active and aren't even breaking a sweat, you're not pushing hard enough. And don't be snooty or shy about sweating. Sweating just means the body is working efficiently to try to cool off. Not sweating is harmful.

Movement is not supposed to be uncomfortable — that's a signal that it's not being done right. For now, just understand that movement needs to done on a regular basis, sustained long enough to burn fat, and be comfortable. Simply moving is easier to remember than measuring heart rate, figuring out target heart rate, and deciding exactly what type of exercise you should do.

Now that you've taken a deep breath and relaxed, let's talk about "dieting." Dieting is so wrought with negative feelings and thoughts that interfere with our success in losing weight, that we must eliminate it forever. Not a bad thought, huh? So, why do we usually feel nervous about that thought? Feeling nervous is normal. We've been taught to believe that we can't lose weight without dieting and, conversely, that if we are not dieting when we are trying to lose weight, then we are doing something "bad."

Nothing is further from the truth. Most overweight people are on a diet, have just gotten off a diet, or have been on many diets before. Most thin people are not on a diet, are not even thinking about dieting, and have never been on a diet to lose weight. Who do you think is more expert at being thin? Yep.

So, in getting leaner, doesn't it make sense to study thin people who don't diet? What do they do? What do they eat? How do they manage their weight?

Not dieting makes some logical sense. It makes life more enjoyable. As you learn more about the advantages of eliminating dieting from your life, you can relax.

Not dieting doesn't mean not caring about your nutrition or what you eat. It does mean that you:

- Believe you can eat whatever you want whenever you want.

- Let go of the belief that there are "good" foods or "bad" foods. All food is good. Some food is good because it is nutritious, some because it tastes good; some food is both nutritious and tastes good.

- Don't have to eat anything that you don't like and enjoy.

- Don't eliminate your favorite foods from your life.

- Don't count calories, fats, carbohydrates, or anything else.

- Take a casual approach to eating — relax, think about what you really want to eat and eat it.

"How can I lose weight this way?" you might ask. Not only can you lose fat with this perspective, but also, it is by far, the most lasting way to do it. In the remaining chapters we will go into more detail about each of the subjects that are important to successful weight loss. There will be simple instructions for each of these. By the end of the book, you will be equipped to calmly achieve fitness for life, while focusing on more important things, such as inner peace, happiness, good relationships, play, enjoyable work, laughter, and ACCEPTANCE.

Chapter 2 Tidbits

- The basics of successful weight loss are physical activity, nutrition, and eliminating dieting.

- Exercise is just another form of movement. More movement equals more fat burned.

- You don't need to measure, weigh, or count to have good nutrition.

- All food is good. It can be good because it's nutritious, because it tastes good, or both.

- We can learn more about how to lose weight successfully by studying how naturally thin people go about their lives than we can by reading diet books.

My "Mind Over Fat Matters" Notes

What I want to remember:

What I want to do:

How this will enrich my life:

Chapter 3

Moving to the Music of Life:

The Role of Exercise in

Successful Weight Loss

We've already generally discussed the biological or physiological side of exercise as it relates to burning fat. Here's a quick review in case you think you forgot.

Those people who move more in general in their lives burn more calories than those who are sedentary. You can increase your metabolism or fat-burning rate by adding regular, sustained exercise to your lifestyle. This exercise or movement can be any activity you like that makes you breathe deeply, but won't make you run out of breath.

In this chapter we will concern ourselves with the psychological side of things. You accept that exercise helps to make you a better fat burner. You've wanted to exercise regularly to lose weight but just the thought sends you running the other way, or you've tried numerous times to start a good exercise program, only to quit after little time. The time between your exercise attempts is much longer than the time you've spent exercising, so you haven't changed much in the weight-loss area.

First of all, throw any guilt about not exercising or giving up, out the window. It's a useless emotion for us. Contrary to what adults taught us as children, guilt does not motivate you to do better. If guilt motivated, how many more things would you have achieved in life? It won't work this time, either, to riddle yourself with guilt over the past. Besides, you didn't have the right information about making it work. You hadn't been helped to deal with the psychological barriers that were getting in your way. You behaved normally if we consider that you are a human being (imperfect), and considering the approach you were taking, your reaction was the correct one.

What was the approach you were taking? You expected perfection, believed it should be easy, used guilt to motivate, picked exercises that you didn't like, exercised too strenuously, and exercised for only one reason — to lose weight. Your approach may have included more than the above or you may have only used some of these methods. No matter, even if you were guilty of just one of these, you were at a disadvantage. Did you catch that one? I used the word "guilty." If you caught it, you are on your way to successfully getting rid of the burden of guilt. If you didn't catch it, don't feel guilty (ha!).

I like to talk about perfection. I got a lot of practice with it while treating eating disorders for 15 years. "Perfection" is not a helpful word. As fallible humans, we're doomed from the start if we expect perfection. Imperfection is precisely what gives us our individuality. Humans are interesting when they are not perfect. Just look around next time you're in the mall. No one is perfect, not even the people you may believe have everything. Life is simpler when you accept this fact. You can remove a huge burden from your life by letting go of the notion of perfection. If you want to spend more time feeling good, laughing, smiling, and experiencing the joy in life, vow to give up expecting perfection. But be careful not to expect to be perfect at giving up perfection!

Enough said. You'll learn as you go along how letting go of the notion of perfection can be empowering. Now, let's learn how to start exercising for life.

Stop using the word "exercise." The word "exercise" has too many negative things associated with it and the word implies that only certain activities qualify as "exercise." Try to catch yourself when using the word and consciously say, "Moving is all I want to do. Any form of movement is good for the life I want." The more you catch yourself and replace "exercise" with "movement," the sooner you'll feel calmer with the thought of it.

Take the time to choose forms of movement that fit who you are. You don't have to use the same form of movement for the rest of your life. You can change things whenever you want. Like to dance? Dance any way you want, to anything you want. Do you like dancing free form in only your underwear to the music of the radio? Then do it! Of course, you should take into consideration any physical limitations you may have. A broken ankle does not preclude movement just because you can't move on your feet. Putting off moving until you heal isn't going to help. This is where creativity comes in. A former patient of mine, who had some foot problems, learned that she could move her arms to music and just lift her legs at the knees. This still got her heart moving and burned more fat than doing nothing but sitting and watching TV.

If you really dislike something, don't do it. It doesn't matter if everyone else does it. Don't jog just because most people jog when they're trying to lose weight. Don't join a gym or exercise with someone else if it is not you. This may sound like the opposite of much of the advice about exercise you have heard before. Don't sweat the small stuff. Accepting that you're not the type to enroll in aerobic classes and quickly looking for activities you find more comfortable to think about will give better results. I went to a gym for years but never liked it. I wanted to walk in, work out and get out. It delayed me to make small talk with people that wanted to socialize more than exercise. Most of my friends feel they need the environment of a gym and others exercising to keep motivated. I just wasn't like most of my friends. Why push it? I finally got smart and set up a simple workout room at home. I've been moving regularly in my little room for years now. It's definitely me!

Start slow. There are two reasons for this. Some people think they have to be able to move as quickly and as long as they see others move during exercising. They don't think about the fact that they may not be as fit as the other person who has been exercising regularly for some time. By starting at your own fitness level (even if that means moving at what seems like a snail's pace) you will gradually progress. Setting deadlines won't help either. It's too much pressure and usually leads to quitting, feeling exhausted, disappointed, and defeated. Instead, if you think of moving like you think of brushing your teeth (you do it regularly without hardly thinking about it), it becomes a habit and one you don't like to go without (like not being able to brush all day).

The second reason to start slowly is a psychological one. The brain has a difficult time taking big steps. The more difficult or uncomfortable it anticipates something to be, the more resistant it will be to it. Translation: you'll quit in short order. Think of a certain goal. Ask yourself if the thought of this goal sounds comfortable. If it doesn't, make the goal smaller. Keep doing this until the goal is small enough to feel easily achievable.

For example, Karen wanted to start a walking program. She had read that she should walk 30 minutes each day in order to lose weight. The thought of walking for 30 minutes felt overwhelming to her but she ignored the signal. She had never liked walking but it was the exercise rage and it was supposed to be "the best way to lose weight." Karen did walk 30 minutes the first day but it felt cumbersome the entire time and she was winded. She was bored and felt time passing at an unbearably slow pace. She was exhausted in the end and for the next few days suffered with painful muscle soreness. Too sore to walk the next day, she told herself she would get back into it after the soreness let up. Karen didn't admit it to herself but she knew she wouldn't continue. Karen eventually became a regular "mover" but it didn't happen until she listened to her brain. She liked dancing so she started modern dance lessons. The dance lessons were fun. She wanted to keep dancing because it felt good and a nice side effect was fat loss.

Put weight loss at the bottom of your list of reasons for why you want to move more. There are other benefits to being more active than just fat loss. Here are some from people I've worked with: "To live longer and better"; "To strengthen my heart"; "To get in touch with nature"; "To give me some alone time"; "To help me think more creatively"; "To have fun"; "To feel like a child again"; "To get a break from responsibilities"; "To watch my muscles get more toned"; "To get stronger"; "To be able to keep up with my husband or wife or kids." It's easy to come up with more reasons if you think about it.

Work with your thinking. Remember your brain can be your biggest obstacle or your best friend. If you don't work with your thinking, you're allowing the brain to work against you. Learning to think more realistically takes some focus at first but the changes will be permanent and well worth the effort. In Section II, we will get into more detail about conquering psychological barriers and you'll learn exactly what to do to change defeating thinking.

Have a playful attitude. Remember what it felt like to be a child? Your major job was to play. Each day was just another adventure, another play day. Sure, most of us had some serious things we had to do sometimes, but we just looked forward to being free of it so we could get back to our main purpose: playing. What happened? Where is it written that adults can't play? When are adults allowed to play? As adults, we approach life as serious business. Play, if we allow ourselves to have it, is rationed and has to be earned.

Well, I'm here to say, "There's no law that prohibits adults from having a playful attitude all the time. It's okay. It won't make you irresponsible or lazy. What it *will* do is make life fun, give fewer wrinkles, improve your relationships, improve your creativity, make you more active, and make exercise pleasant. When you take a playful approach to life, you view exercise as an opportunity to play instead of as a burdensome responsibility. You'll feel that you *want* to move, rather than that you *should* move. Another advantage of this perspective is that you won't want anything to get in the way of your playing time. The more you play, the more fat is burned!

So, the words to remember are "move" and "play." They can make the difference between success and failure.

Chapter 3 Tidbits

- Feeling guilty and trying to be perfect will not motivate you.

- Children are active because they think of activity as play. Play is fun; it feels good. Forget about exercise — just play.

- Children don't all like to play in the same way. Be sure your play activity fits who you are. It must be movement you enjoy. Nobody else has to like it.

- Forget about weight loss. The object is to move and have fun at it. If you move, you'll likely lose weight.

My "Mind Over Fat Matters" Notes

What I want to remember:

What I want to do:

How this will enrich my life:

Chapter 4

Nutrition Made Easy:

How to Eat Well Without

Trying So Hard

Let's face it. Successful weight management is dependent on a lifestyle of healthy nutrition. The problem is that nutrition, like exercise, turns many people off. Some people think nutrition means no taste. Why would someone want to eat foods with no taste the rest of their lives?

We think that to know about nutrition means learning complicated facts about health, types of food, fat, sugar, vitamin and mineral content, and measurements that we can't figure out. How much is a gram? How much is a serving? Which foods are high in calcium or vitamin A? What nutrients are in spinach? Am I getting enough fiber if I eat 12 grams a day? No wonder we shy away from nutrition! It's too hard and no fun at all.

It's logical to want to stay away from things that are complex, not fun, and that make us feel insecure about our ability to master them. It's normal. Everybody's seeking to have a happy life free of stress, fears, and excessive work. The old nutrition advice doesn't make us feel free of these.

Eating well takes little attention and time, and eating should taste good, be simple, and be relaxing. Actually, I prefer the term "eating well" to the word "nutrition." "Nutrition" sounds like it deals only with the specific nutrient content of foods and it sounds complicated to boot. On the other hand, "eating well" allows room for other information about eating, such as food groups, fiber, time of eating, snacking, calorie-filled foods that are not noticeable, and food colors.

Let's breeze through all you need to know about nutrition. Nutrition is simply all the good things contained in foods, which, in turn, are healthy for our bodies and minds. Some of these things are vitamins, minerals, and fats. Enough. We can have good nutrition without getting a Ph.D. in it.

Here's all we have to know:

There are five food groups:

Protein Group — chicken, beef, pork, fish, other types of meat and poultry, eggs, and nuts, to name a few protein items.

Fruit and Vegetable Group — oranges, kiwis, bananas, avocados, apples, tomatoes, etc. (all fruit); potatoes, broccoli, lettuce, corn, peppers, etc. (all vegetables).

Bread/Cereal Group — all breads, rolls, biscuits, pasta, and grains, such as oatmeal, rye, wheat, brown rice, millet, and breakfast cereals.

Dairy Group — here we have the cheeses, milks, yogurt, and ice cream (yum!).

Treat Group — I don't think I have to tell you what goes in this group. Some treats have a lot of nutrition, some don't. It's all in what makes you feel all warm and fuzzy.

Typically, the less processing the food has gone through before it gets to our mouths, the better. Raw fruits and vegetables are better for us than frozen. Frozen fruits and vegetables are better than canned. Canned foods have been through the most processing, which decreases their nutritional value. Whole grains (wheat, rye, brown rice) are better for us than the whiter kind (it's whiter because the good stuff, which is on the outside, has been removed).

Anything prepared with fat (fried, buttered, sauces and spreads, in general) will have more calories than if it were broiled, baked, or grilled. Yellow cheeses usually have more fat than white cheeses. Skin on chicken is fat. It doesn't mean that you can't eat it, just know what it is. Red meat usually has more fat (not taking into consideration how it was prepared) than chicken, fish, or other white meats. The more expensive red meats are usually fattier. That's because we like our meats tender, and fat makes meat tender.

By eating something daily from each food group (except the treats group, which is included more for the mind than for the body), you will provide your body with more nutrition than most people get. You could get compulsive about nutrition, but unless it's fun and comfortable, you'll sacrifice other important things in life and probably quit after awhile anyway. Casually focusing on having something from the bread/cereal group, the fruit/vegetable group, the meat group, and the dairy group each day will supply most of the nutrients you need. Throwing in a treat for good measure is also wise.

Good nutrition is colorful. It has reds, greens, yellows, and purples, to name a few. A plate without much nutrition tends to look bland, mostly earth tones and whites. The only color in a typical fast food hamburger is the lonely slice of tomato. The nutrition-challenged iceberg lettuce only has a hint of green. Here are some simple questions to ask yourself when you look at your plate: "Is there much color here? How many colors have I eaten today?"

Figuring out normal serving sizes can make you want to pull your hair out. Sure, most food packaging has labeling showing their recommended serving size, but what kind of serving size is it? Have you ever measured a serving size from one of these labels? Why does a packet of pasta that has enough for just three people say that it feeds eight? Each serving is supposed to be two ounces or 59 pieces. How much is two ounces and who wants to count out 59 pieces times three? Not me! Knowing what a normal serving size is can be helpful in losing weight, but it doesn't have to be as precise or time-consuming as you might think. Here are some tips on how to serve reasonable amounts without the hassle:

- If the food item has small units or is often cut into small units like corn, peas, cooked rice, peanuts, or beans, think of half a cup, or the amount that would fill a cupped hand. You can use your own personal guide if it is easier for you. Sometimes I'll look at the size of the opening of my fingers if I form a "C" with my hand and serve myself an amount that would form the same size circle on my plate.

- For meats, using the size of the palm of the hand is a good example of a reasonable serving.

- Liquids other than water — such as beer, juices, sodas, and milk — are important because we can easily fool ourselves into thinking that they don't have any calories. The average sugared soda has calories. Plenty of people drink sugared sodas throughout the day as if they were drinking water. At the end of a day, a heavy soda drinker may have added several hundred extra calories to his or her body. If you consider that this person drinks this amount of soda every day, you can see how easily he or she can get fat and wonder how it happened. Packaged fruit juice has a lot more calories than the fresh version and is a lot easier to consume. It's hardly noticeable that any calories have entered your body when you savor your refreshing drink. For our purposes in keeping things simple, one regular-sized glass would be a serving. It's not important to be precise. It won't be "Big Gulp" size or the baby juice glasses they give you at many restaurants.

- Bready foods — like sliced bread, muffins, bagels, and rolls — are easy, too. If the bread is being added to a regular meal, one slice is a reasonable average portion. If it's part of a sandwich, two slices would be the serving size. One bagel or muffin would be an average serving size.

- What about things like ice cream or cookies or candy? Think of an ice cream serving as two scoops. Cookies, if small, three or four, if large, one.

- Some people are used to eating large servings, no sweat. Remember, the brain deals best with small steps. Simply start where you're at (let's say, 10 cookies) and gradually reduce the amount. Go to nine cookies for a while (or nine and a half if the brain is saying it's too big a step), then eight, seven, and so on. Another version of small steps is to substitute something else that's tasty but has less fat or calories. I taught a patient to substitute an apple for one of her cookies. The apple had less fat and calories than the cookie and was bulkier so it had more fiber. It was more nutritious, crunchier, and more color-ful. Sometimes she couldn't finish the apple because it filled her up sooner than the cookie. The end result was that she ended up eating even less than she had set out to eat.

The most important thing is to relax. You can be creative and come up with other methods that work. If the method feels exciting, motivating, and free of anxiety, then congratulations — you've got it! It's also important to remember that if something is not working, it's not working. There's no rea-son to continuing doing it. Instead, use smaller steps or think of something else to try. There are no deadlines here. You're working on the rest of your life and the kinder you are to yourself, the faster it will work.

Chapter 4 Tidbits

- You don't have to know much about nutrition to eat well. Nutrition is simply all the good things contained in foods, which, in turn, are healthy for our bodies and minds.

- Having fun with food is more important than knowing a lot of facts about food.

- If your plate looks colorful, contains foods that taste good and aren't too doctored up (fried, processed, swimming in sauces), you're eating well.

- Relax and enjoy eating!

My "Mind Over Fat Matters" Notes

What I want to remember:

What I want to do:

How this will enrich my life:

Chapter 5

The Four-Letter Word:

The Role of "Diet" in

Successful Weight Loss

"Diet" is today's four-letter word. We use it about as frequently as some of our other "naughty" words. It used to be a normal word with no emotion associated with it: a neutral word. It was simply a description of our food patterns. Later, it actually was seen as a good word. It also came to mean a pattern of eating nutritious foods that led to health or weight loss. Before long, we started using "diet" to mean a food program specifically and intentionally used for losing weight. Diets became fads not much different from other fads, such as Beanie Babies, quiche, Pokémon, baggy pants, and expensive sneakers. There was the Atkins Diet, the Stillman Diet, the Rotation Diet, and the Grapefruit Diet, to name just a few. Some diets, like the Atkins high-protein diet, have made a comeback.

During the 1970s and 1980s — what I call "The Diet Era" — it was almost a status symbol to be on a diet to lose weight. "Oh, no, thank-you. I'm on a diet." "Have you tried the Rotation Diet? It makes you lose a ton of weight!" Dieters would make these statements proudly as if their being on a diet meant they were being good, strong, and responsible. As Americans became more weight conscious, the more dieting became part of our lifestyle. That's good, right?

In our case, it's not a good thing. Many people believe that if something is good, then more is better. It's usually not the case. Losing weight is good, right? It depends on how much we lose, how fast we lose, and its cost. Dieting surely is good. It depends on the type of diet, the number of calories, the nutrients, how long the diet lasts, and what's sacrificed for the sake of following the diet and losing weight.

It was during the "Diet Era" that eating disorders exploded into an epidemic. It was also during this time that Americans on the average started getting fatter — faster! We've ended up with the two extremes.

One of the costs to all of us is that "diet" is no longer a neutral word. "Diet" conjures up thoughts of deprivation, little enjoyment, cravings, having to eat things we don't like, and not being able to eat foods we love. It brings on feelings of anxiety, frustration, resistance, fear, and maybe even anger. Today we still think we should be on a diet and we think it should be easy, but we cringe at the thought of dieting.

The truth is that strict dieting results in weight gain — the opposite of what we want. Of course, most dieters don't know that the dieting is causing their weight gain. Instead, they believe themselves to be to blame because of their lack of control or discipline. Nothing could be further from the truth. The problem is with the diet and the brain's reaction to it.

Your body and, particularly, your brain, are built to help you survive. In fact, the most important thing to your brain is to prevent your destruction. You don't have to do much to survive physically; you're essentially on "autopilot" most of the time. That leaves you free to relax and enjoy life; unless, that is, you interfere with your brain's function to help you survive and, by dieting strictly, you get in its way.

The brain is an expert at knowing what your body needs. Someone who has never dieted has strong communication with his or her brain. If the brain registers that it needs something, it signals us to seek it.

For example, Jane has never been on a diet. She can't remember ever having to think much about food. If she felt like eating something, she ate it. Sometimes she'd feel like having meat, other times fruit would appeal to her. In the morning, she usually wanted something starchy and, at night, she'd feel like having something sweet. When she ate what she wanted, she quickly felt satisfied and went on to other things in her life.

Joyce, on the other hand, started trying diets when she was 15 years old. Usually the diets were low in calories and had many restrictions, particularly about what she could and could not eat. Joyce tried to stay away from some of her favorite foods, such as bread, sweets, and pizza, because she believed they were fattening. In order to stay on the diets, she had to watch what she ate carefully and make sure not to loosen up on any of the restrictions. She'd plan meals or skip them completely whenever possible. Only "diet" foods were allowed in her kitchen and when she had a craving for something, she would try to distract herself from it through any means possible. Despite all her efforts, the longer she was on the diet, the harder it was to stay on it.

Joyce became obsessed with food, sometimes even dreaming about it. She'd anticipate the next opportunity to eat but felt anxious, fearing she would lose control and break the diet. She felt hungry a lot but rarely felt completely satisfied after a meal. Joyce was familiar with what would happen if she let herself eat something she wasn't supposed to eat. Lately, she had secretly been eating compulsively, and eating out with friends was too tempting and frustrating.

I could go on but it's probably clear. Jane's story is short: Jane wants pizza. Jane eats pizza. Jane feels satisfied. Jane continues to enjoy her life.

Joyce's story is long and doesn't have an ending. Joyce wants ice cream. Joyce doesn't eat ice cream. Joyce gets a stronger urge for ice cream. Joyce tries harder not to eat ice cream. Joyce can't get ice cream off her mind. Joyce tries like hell to avoid the ice cream. Joyce is nervous, afraid, and salivating like crazy. Joyce breaks down and eats a half-gallon of ice cream. Joyce feels guilty and mad at herself. Joyce gains weight. Joyce goes on another diet. Everything repeats.

When the brain is fed, it relaxes and focuses on other things. It needs fuel to function and food is its fuel. It can't afford to wait until the fuel tank is completely empty to sound the alarm. When it senses that it's not getting the amount of fuel it needs, it starts to send warnings. However, most people don't know how to read the brain's signals. When you're on a strict diet and you start thinking about food more or getting strong cravings, it's your brain trying to tell you to feed it. It may try to push you to eat particular types of foods if it's lacking in particular nutrients, like craving meat when your body needs some protein.

Most diets, though, are too low in calories to supply your body with the needed fuel. In these cases, the brain's goal is to get you to eat anything with calories. That's usually the foods with the most concentrated calorie-content fats. If your body is highly deprived of calories, it's not going to waste its time trying to get you to eat an apple and some carrots. It's going to point you straight to the mud pie or the fried chicken.

Not knowing that the cravings are attempts from the brain to help, the dieter becomes afraid that she will lose control and break the diet. In an effort to prevent this, she tries harder to follow the diet instead of listening to what her body tells her. The harder she tries, the stronger the signals from her brain to eat. Usually, the brain wins and the dieter succumbs to the cravings or, depending on how long and to what degree she has deprived herself, she binges.

Let's take a closer look at Jane and Joyce's approaches to eating. Jane takes a casual, relaxed approach to her eating life. Her eating is naturally in control; she doesn't have to focus on it. Joyce is uptight about her eating and she sometimes binges. Which way is more likely to result in any weight loss?

Joyce's method can only lead to weight gain or an eating disorder (we will discuss eating disorders in more detail in Chapter 21). There's more. Joyce isn't happy. She's irritable, anxious, and frustrated. In short, she's not having much fun and the quality of her life is being compromised.

Dieting leads to deprivation. In turn, deprivation leads to the brain trying to protect the body by pushing it to eat. The longer the brain is deprived, the bigger the binge is going to be. The bigger and more frequent the binges, the greater the weight gain. It's a well-known fact that dieters usually regain more weight after stopping a diet than they lost while on the diet.

When control of food occurs, not because of a conscious decision to control, but because our body is in balance, we would say it is in "natural control." Natural control looks like this: you sense you want something to eat (it could be due to hunger or just a yearning). You think of what specifically you want (let's say, jelly beans) and allow yourself to have it. You get exactly what you want, jelly beans, and happily savor every mouthful. At some point, your brain sends a message, "I don't want any more." You stop eating and go on to something else.

When you're in natural control, you don't have to think much about eating. You go with the flow and let your brain direct you automatically. There's no need to try to figure out when enough is enough. You let your brain be the guide — it's the expert!

Trying to control eating leads to loss of control. What a "Catch-22!" That's the way it is, though. It's how we are wired. Humans know little about how the brain works, especially when we consider all its capabilities. It's an amazing machine and we're lucky to have it.

Unfortunately, too many people have needlessly suffered trying to follow the wrong advice about losing weight — blaming themselves when they fail at it. The good news is that it's simple to regain natural control over food. We all have the ability for natural control of eating. After all, we weren't born overeating. As babies, like with other animals, our brain told us when we needed food and we cried to communicate it. As we got older, we got better at communicating it until we were able to get our own food.

What's the bottom line? Get rid of the word "diet" from your vocabulary; let go of dieting. Only when you let go of dieting can you regain natural control. Doesn't it feel good to know that you never have to diet again? But, how do you do this?

The first step toward gaining natural control is to stop dieting. Scary thought? The first thing my patients would say when I would give them the good news was, "But if I stop dieting and let myself eat what I want, I'll totally lose control and won't be able to stop eating. I'll get fat!"

It is understandable that the idea of stopping dieting would conjure up these types of thoughts. After all, it has probably been a long time since you felt what it was like to be in natural control of your eating. If you think carefully, you'll realize that was when you weren't on a strict diet. You haven't lost the ability to be in natural control of your eating — you've just forgotten how to do it. The remainder of this book is designed to help you regain this ability. You can start by realizing that "Diet" is a destructive four-letter word.

Chapter 5 Tidbits

- The brain is an expert at knowing what your body needs. If we listen, it will tell us exactly what we need to eat.

- Most people who diet are overweight.

- "Diet" is a bad word and dieting is destructive. Come up with words that your brain will embrace instead of resist, and with methods that will be fun to follow. When the brain is happy, it never stops helping us to achieve our goals.

- We are all born with natural control over food. Strict dieting can get in the way by leading to loss of control and overeating. Eliminating dieting helps us "get back to nature" and feel in control again.

- The first step toward natural control of food is to stop dieting.

My "Mind Over Fat Matters" Notes

What I want to remember:

What I want to do:

How this will enrich my life:

Part II

Conquering Psychological

Barriers

We all have psychological barriers — emotional conflicts or fears that are part of personality and lead to resistance and failure with efforts to control weight. We wouldn't be human if we didn't have them. The newborn has a clean slate until the moment he or she enters the world. For the rest of its life, the child's experiences will affect everything he or she thinks, feels, and does. The fact that I'm writing at this moment, how I'm writing, and how I feel about my writing, has been shaped by all that has happened to me before this moment.

It's always been hard for me to get myself to sit and write. I went through graduate school and earned a Ph.D. with this problem. Obviously, I've done enough writing to accomplish some things and I've worked to prevent the problem from controlling my life, but it is one of my biggest psychological barriers in life. Why do I resist writing when I have such a strong desire to do it? It's not totally clear to me, but I know that ever since I can remember, I've thought that I wasn't a good writer.

Through the years, I've become a better writer, but the monster still likes to show its ugly head from time to time. "It's too hard to write," it says. "You won't be able to express your thoughts well enough for people to understand or be interested. Besides, you don't feel that well today. Your neck hurts too much to be able to do a good job. You haven't fed the squirrels yet and there's some gardening you need to do. You can do that first and write later." The monster is clever.

Psychological barriers wall us off from things we want. I've never known a person who didn't have at least one nice, juicy, barrier to their dreams in life. They usually come from our childhood experiences, such as the child whose parent said he or she would never amount to anything, or the woman whose cousin used to make fun of her nose when they were kids. Sometimes psychological barriers can stem from things that happen in adulthood. Going through a difficult break-up or having a serious accident can build walls that make us want to run from things that, at one time, were no problem. So it is with managing our weight.

Psychological barriers can vary from person to person. While one person's psychological barrier might be his perfectionism, another may fail time and time again because of his problem with anger. Some other psychological barriers include depression, anxiety, inability to delay gratification (wait for the reward), and low self-esteem.

In Part II of *Mind Over Fat Matters*, we will delve into the more common psychological barriers to losing weight, keeping it off, and having natural control of eating.

Chapter 6

Get a Life: Life Vs. Weight

It's simple, really. The higher the quality of our lives, the happier we will be. The most essential ingredients in quality of life are health, relationships, food, shelter, love, and self-esteem. Any major problem in any of these areas and the quality of our lives goes down, and so does our happiness. That's why some of the major stressors in life are the death of a loved one, a serious or chronic illness, divorce, losing a job, and depression.

When people say, "Get a life," what do they mean? They mean, "Seek some meaningful purpose in life." It means we should take care of ourselves, form good relationships, eat well, work well, play well, and have love in our lives. We have quality of life when we have all these things in balance.

Too often, people allow their weight-loss goals to supersede the quality of their lives. Losing weight becomes central to their existence. More important things are compromised, sometimes even sacrificed, for thinness. Sadly, I've encountered plenty of folks who would ignore their relationships, even to the degree of avoiding sex with their partner, because of focus on weight and appearance.

Here again, our original good intentions are somehow lost in all the overwhelming details of dieting. Why do we want to be thin in the first place? We believe that in the end it will make us happier because it will improve the quality of our lives. Somewhere along the way, we lose sight of our primary goal and, when we lose it, we can't achieve it.

What's the answer? We need to keep our priorities straight. Quality of life and all that it entails needs to be at the top of our list again. Bettering our quality of life needs to be the reason we pursue other goals, including controlling our weight. By doing all the things that will achieve weight loss, but that will not get in the way of our true happiness in life, we accomplish both. We should work on our bodies to live, not live to work on our bodies.

So, before you even begin to learn the how-tos of *Mind Over Fat Matters,* ask yourself, "What's more important to me? Is the most important thing to me being the "right" weight, getting approval from others, or looking a certain way? Are these things more important than my happiness, peace, and health?" If so, disappointment is likely to surface again. On the other hand, if you realize that there are more important things in life than weight, and you're going to give those things priority (while still playfully learning how to be the leanest, healthiest person you can be), you're ready for success and a whole lot of fun. You've reached "GO."

Chapter 6 Tidbits

- The greater the quality of your life, the happier you will be.

- Putting weight and appearance first in life only leads to disappointment, low self-esteem, unhappiness, and makes it next to impossible to reach your weight goals.

- When you don't sweat the small stuff, you keep your priorities straight and, if you enjoy life, the rest will come.

- Get a life!

My "Mind Over Fat Matters" Notes

What I want to remember:

What I want to do:

How this will enrich my life:

Chapter 7

Rules: Your Worst Enemies

Rules are all-or-nothing expectations of ourselves that allow us no flexibility. Rules say such things as, "I will never gain weight again. I'll always eat exactly what is on my diet. I must never eat sweets or fried foods." Rules don't say such things as, "I'm going to strive to eat more fruits and vegetables every day. I'm going to work at increasing my movement level so that I can learn to be a more active person." No. Rules say, "Thou shall not…" or "Thou shall always…" There may be a proper place for rules, like those set up for nuclear power plants to prevent catastrophes, but they have no place in our eating world.

When you're dealing with eating, you have to work with the physiology and psychology of your body. Here, rules upset the preprogrammed balance and break down the system. To give an extreme example (but a real one), someone with anorexia is slowly starving her body and mind. As the anorexic deprives her body, it slowly starts to malfunction by slowing its metabolism, losing vital elements essential to her body's survival and, eventually, even causing brain damage. This is only a short list of the potentially destructive side effects of anorexia.

Most diets are made up of rules. You may eat meat and fats but no carbohydrates, for example. Even if the diet is meant to be flexible, often the dieter turns any guidelines into rules. It's an attempt to be extra "good" and speed up the weight-loss process, but it makes the "new and improved diet" less effective than the original. As a matter of fact, it makes the diet ineffective.

Rules lead to "psychological deprivation." With physiological deprivation, such as a lack of food or water, if we don't have the food or water, we eventually die. We won't die if we're psychologically deprived, but it will make our lives hell. When we're psychologically deprived, we're refusing to give ourselves something we like a lot, but we don't need it to live. If we're not allowed to have water, our days are numbered, but, if we're not allowed pizza again, we'll continue living. Our lives won't be as enjoyable without our golden, cheesy disc of delight, but we won't die. We have only been psychologically deprived.

Another way to look at psychological deprivation is by thinking of your least favorite food — something you really hate. A commonly despised food is spinach (if you happen to like spinach, then substitute something else). Let's say someone (who had total control over our lives) said, "You may *never* have spinach again." Is that music I hear? No more spinach, you say? Sure, no problem. You don't like spinach so you'd consider it a favor (maybe a miracle) if you never had to set eyes on the green, slimy stuff again. No psychological deprivation here.

Now, let's say that same person said, "You may *never* have pizza again — ever, ever, ever." That one person who likes spinach probably hates pizza, but you get the idea. Substitute your most favorite food (ice cream, chocolate, bread, jelly beans, macaroni and cheese, maybe). Now think of spending the rest of your life without being able to eat your special treat. You may watch other people eating it; you can see it in stores, but you can't taste it ever again. Not so comfortable now, huh? Do you feel a little anxious, maybe even fearful or irritated? Are you picturing the most beautiful specimen of pizza ever known to man? Your mouth is watering. You want pizza right NOW! It's hard to think of anything else. Voila! You have just experienced some psychological deprivation.

With psychological deprivation come feelings of tension, preoccupation, and being out of control — a pull towards the "taboo" food like you've never felt before. The longer the deprivation, the stronger the pull, until it's humanly impossible to resist any longer. At this point, you break down and eat the pizza, ice cream, or bread like there's no tomorrow.

Let's take a closer look at the psychology of rules. Rules work on us in a cyclical manner. In order to describe best how rules work, I'll use an analogy. I often use religion as an analogy for the cyclical nature of rules (note: religion is used only to best demonstrate a point and for no other purpose. I grew up Catholic so I will use what I learned as a child for my example. I'm sure there are other concepts that would work as well).

In most Christian religions, there are a set of laws that are similar to rules in that they are all-or-nothing. These laws are The Ten Commandments. The

Ten Commandments say such things as, "Thou shall not kill." "Thou shall not steal." "Thou shall honor thy mother and thy father." They do not say, "Try not to steal too much in your lifetime." "Try not to kill more than once or twice." "If you dishonor thy mother and father occasionally, it's no big deal." No. They clearly say, "Thou shall *not...*" ever, or "Thou *shall...*" always. If the laws are broken, even once, it is supposed to mean we have sinned. We've done something wrong or bad.

Now let's compare that to a rule we'll make about chocolate chip cookies." Our rule says, "I must never eat chocolate chip cookies. If I take just one bite of a chocolate chip cookie, I have broken my rule; I've done something wrong or bad."

In our religion example, when we're enticed to do something that goes against The Ten Commandments, we usually refer to this as "temptation." With rules, we feel psychologically deprived of the cookies and are more focused on them. Now, instead of chocolate chip cookies being just cookies, they are COOKIES! They are bigger than life. They're thick, soft, and chewy cookies that make our mouths water uncontrollably and seem to have power over us.

But, wait. We have a rule that says we must never eat chocolate chip cookies. Because we have this rule and our psychological deprivation is pushing us to have the cookies, we must tighten up our rule to prevent a breakdown. "No, no, no. I must not have any cookies. I'll try to distract myself, maybe go exercise or something. I'll just grit my teeth and bare it."

When we tighten our rules, we only psychologically deprive ourselves even more, which makes us focus on the cookies more. The push to have the cookies gets stronger and stronger until we can't control it any longer. It's not our fault. Our brain just doesn't work well with rules.

Suddenly we find ourselves in a feeding frenzy. This isn't a situation where we calmly sit down and slowly savor our cookies. No, we eat them fast, as if it's our last chance to have chocolate chip cookies. Not only that, but we barely taste each one before we're shoving the next one in our mouth. We feel out of control and we are. We can't seem to find satisfaction as we continue to eat, until we can't fit any more cookies in our stomach or someone walks in on us (we don't want to look like a pig, after all).

In the end, we've eaten more chocolate chip cookies than we ever did before we set a rule about them. This is compulsive eating, or binging. It can happen to any one. It's not how much we eat that determines whether we're eating compulsively or not — it's how we feel while we're eating. Remember, when we have natural control over food, we are calm, content, and we slowly savor food. When we eat compulsively, we're tense, we feel out of control, and we barely taste our food. When we have natural control, we stop eating automatically after eating a reasonable amount of food. When we're compulsively eating, we can't stop until our body won't hold any more or some other external event forces us to stop.

Let's picture a large circle. Better yet, take out a piece of paper and a pencil and draw a large circle. This circle represents the process we go through psychologically and behaviorally when we try to set rules about our eating. At the top of the circle is our rule: "I must never eat chocolate chip cookies." Write this rule at the top and outside of the circle. Using our religion example, our rule would be equivalent to a Commandment because it is black and white. There is no flexibility in it. So, on the inside of the circle and directly opposite of our rule, write the word "Commandment."

Now, draw an arrow leading away from our rule and another from the Commandment following the circle. At the end of the arrow leading from the rule, write the word "Urge." After the arrow leading from "Commandment," write the word "Temptation." So, our rule leads to an urge for chocolate chip cookies because it has psychologically deprived us and, therefore, we want the cookies even more. Because of our psychological deprivation, cookies are no longer "cookies," but, rather, "COOKIES!" In the religion example, the Commandment is followed by the temptation to do what the Commandment says not to do.

Continuing on, draw arrows from the words "Urge" and "Temptation," following the circle around, and write in the words "Binge" (following "Urge") and "Sin" (following "Temptation"). After we've made a rule, and because we've been psychologically deprived, sooner or later, we binge. The binge would be equivalent to "sin" in our religion example. When we break a Commandment, we are said to have sinned. When we sin, we are supposed to feel guilt and remorse. When we break a rule, we binge. When we binge or eat compulsively, we feel guilt and remorse. So, after the arrows leading from "Sin" and "Binge," plug in the words "Remorse" and "Guilt," respectively.

Now we have the Commandment leading to "Temptation," which leads to "Sin" and then "Remorse." In the case of our eating, we have the Rule leading to an "Urge," which leads to a "Binge" that leads to "Guilt."

When I was growing up, if we sinned and felt remorse, we could go to confession. In confession, we could be cleansed of our sins. We could essentially start over, vowing to abide by The Commandments again. As I remember, the priest would say something like, "Now go and sin no more." The implication was to go and follow the laws of the church again, to the letter, for the rest of our lives.

What is it that dieters do after they've broken their rules and lost control? Typically, the dieter sooner or later vows to follow her rules again, to the letter, from then on. This is the dieter's intention. She's serious; she is really going to do it this time. So, following the words "Remorse" and "Guilt," we have arrows leading to our "Vow" to follow laws again and "Intention" to follow our food rule perfectly from now on. With our "Intention" in place, this time it's really going to work. Unfortunately, this only starts the cycle all over again. By trying to strengthen our rule by intending to follow it perfectly again, we only deprive ourselves even more, which leads to greater urges to eat the "forbidden" food, which leads to more breaking of the rules through loss of control of our eating, more guilt, and on and on and on — indefinitely.

So what do we do? Who wants to go around in circles endlessly? I've seen many people on merry-go-rounds for years, even decades, until they finally discover why all their efforts and intentions haven't worked.

The only way to break the never-ending cycle of rules and compulsive eating is to let go of rules. Note that I didn't say, "Break the rules." Breaking rules happens as a result of having rules in the first place. If we don't have a rule about chocolate chip cookies, and we eat a cookie, we've done nothing wrong. We could eat an entire bag of cookies — no sin, no guilt.

"Okay, I see some logic in what you've said," you may think. "But if I let go of my rules, I'll eat and eat and never be able to stop."

Good thinking. The reason you get this image when you consider letting go of rules is because of the psychological deprivation you know is there. The longer you tell yourself you can't have something you want, the greater your psychological deprivation becomes.

So, are we doomed to be fat whether we have rules or not? No. The good news is that the opposite is also true. If you've been psychologically deprived and you now have no rules, psychological deprivation decreases until it disappears. When it's gone, you return to a state of natural control over food like you had before you ever started having rules.

How does that happen? When you let go of rules you're telling your brain that you can have chocolate chip cookies whenever you want; you can have as many cookies as you desire. At first, your brain says, "Hallelujah! I'm free. Step aside; I'm going straight for the cookies." You'll sit, you'll eat cookies, and you may eat more cookies in one sitting than you ever did before having rules. Or, you may eat chocolate chip cookies every day for a week. If you truly let go and calmly savor the cookies, your brain will start realizing that cookies are always going to be available and no one is going to take them away again. There's no need to eat the whole bag because you can change your mind whenever you want. You can go back to the cookies tomorrow, in an hour, in five minutes, if you feel like it. Now cookies are no longer COOKIES, but normal, everyday, tasty, chocolate chip cookies. Your brain starts saying, "That was good but I think I've had enough for now. Let's do something else." The controls are back with the expert — your brain!

Sure, at first you may overeat, but you have to take responsibility for your psychological deprivation, do what is necessary to heal, and accept the time it takes to heal. Besides, your choice is between overeating that gradually subsides and disappears, or compulsive eating and dieting for the rest of your life. Which approach is more likely to result in weight loss and a life of weight control?

This is a good time to explain the difference between overeating and compulsive eating. When we overeat, we are simply eating more calories than our body needs to do everything it has to do for that day. When we eat compulsively, not only are we eating more than we need, but we're tense while we eat, we eat rapidly, we barely focus on the food, we feel out of control, and we eat attempting to get rid of uncomfortable feelings like anxiety, loneliness, and anger. The overeater enjoys eating. There's no joy in compulsive eating.

Imagine for a minute that Thanksgiving is nearing. Traditionally your family has a big Thanksgiving dinner and Uncle Joe is always invited. This year is no different. A week before the dinner, Uncle Joe is looking forward to the big family dinner. He excitedly thinks about all the great foods he will be able to eat and all the fun he's going to have. You, on the other hand, may be dreading the day because you'll have to confront the large amounts of foods you like so much and but have been on your diet's no-no list. You're afraid you won't be able to control yourself. You may even try to prepare by exercising more and dieting to try to lose some weight before the dreaded day. You start thinking up strategies of how you'll avoid taboo foods and stay in control. You'll eat no bread or dessert, you say — only white, skinless turkey for you, and only tiny servings.

All along, Uncle Joe is just going about his life as usual except for the anticipation of a good time at Thanksgiving dinner. Thanksgiving Day arrives. Uncle Joe starts his day like any other. He'll eat what he usually eats for breakfast and just focuses on getting to dinner on time.

You? Well, you need to try to compensate ahead of time in case you mess up at dinner. You don't eat breakfast; you may exercise, making an attempt to be at a caloric deficit before dinner. Good strategy!

Dinnertime finally arrives. Everyone is sitting at the dinner table. Uncle Joe is laughing, conversing — having a good old time. He's relaxed and thinking only of the present moment. You're tense, having a hard time keeping your mind off all the luscious, mouth-watering food in front of you. You anxiously remind yourself that you can't eat all those fattening things. You can't laugh and play along with everyone because your brain's focused on all that food of which it's been deprived.

Uncle Joe eats everything he wants to eat. He comments about how good it is. He savors his food, while, at the same time, he's able to continue focusing on other things. He's enjoying the atmosphere, the conversations, the jokes, and the wonderful food smells.

You eat, too, but you're feeling out of control. You find yourself eating those very things you told yourself you wouldn't eat. You're not able to stop at the quantities for which you set rules. You can't think of anything else but the food and how you can't stop.

Both you and Uncle Joe stop eating. He, when his body tells him he's full; you, when you can't fit anything else in and you're too embarrassed to be seen eating anymore. Uncle Joe has eaten a lot of food and so have you.

After eating, Uncle Joe retires to an easy chair, loosens his belt, takes a deep sigh and says, "Boy, that was g-o-o-d!" He sits back to relax, converse, and laugh some more. You, on the other hand, also feel terribly full, but you're feeling very tense about it. You're worrying about gaining weight and beating yourself up about eating too much. You're focusing so much on what you have done that you can't pay attention to much else, least of all, partaking in the good time Uncle Joe and the rest of the dinner guests are having. You might already be planning your strategy for compensating for your eating. "Tomorrow I'll start my diet again and this time I'll really stick to it."

After eating, the overeater feels full, very full, but that's it. He is able to stay relaxed and confident that things will get right back to normal soon enough. The dieter feels like she is going to explode. She's extremely anxious and afraid, as if eating too much was the worst thing she could have done. But it's not the end of the world and the overeater knows that. The overeater knows that his body has his best interest in mind and will steer him in the right direction. He trusts his body and listens to it.

In the book by Clarissa Pinkola Estes, *Women Who Run With the Wolves,* she tries to teach women that they are filled with instincts that are good. Estes sees these instincts as a woman's wildish nature and advises women to listen to and be guided in life by these instincts or senses of intuition. Through one of her many creative analogies, Estes compares life to a smorgasbord of food laid out on an endless series of tables. Most people, she says, approach life as though they were rapidly walking along the tables, saying excitedly, "Oh! I would really like to have one of those, and one of that, and some of this other thing." We make choices simply because the thing just happened to be right in front of our noses at that instant. "...the longer we gaze at it, the more compelling it becomes." However, "'When we are connected to the instinctual self, ...we say to ourselves, "What am I hungry for?"'

When you approach food, you need to look and listen inside. Ask yourself, "What do I really want right now?" It doesn't matter what it is. If your brain is telling you it wants to eat something salty, something sweet, something crunchy, meaty, smooth, whatever, you need to not give it a second thought. Instead, you should go get what your brain tells you it wants as soon as possible. And don't try to fool the brain with some inferior version of what it's asking for. Choosing a bargain brand ice cream because it's cheaper when your brain wants Ben and Jerry's is only going to end with your eating the bargain brand, Ben and Jerry's, and maybe other stuff in between. If it's Ben and Jerry's the brain wants, it's Ben and Jerry's that's going to satisfy the brain. Don't fight it — your brain knows better than you what it needs.

Another thing to remember is that the reason why your brain wants something in particular to eat is not important. There are two reasons to eat food. One: you're hungry. Two: you want it. When you're hungry, you need to eat to satisfy a physiological need your body is experiencing. When you simply want something, you need to eat to satisfy a psychological need.

Most diet books will tell you to avoid eating when you're not hungry. First of all, people who have been dieting for a long time have trouble figuring out if they're really hungry. Second, trying to figure this out when you have trouble sensing hunger only induces anxiety. Anxiety makes it harder to figure out if you're hungry. And third, when you can't figure out if you're really hungry, you don't want to make a mistake, so you assume that you're not hungry and try not to eat. This increases your preoccupation with eating until you end up breaking down and eating compulsively — something you wouldn't have done if you had just gone ahead and eaten regardless of the reason for wanting to do so.

Here's an interesting fact. Eating what you want, even when you're not hungry, decreases cravings to eat when you're not hungry. That is, if you eat what you want whenever you want it, you will find that you get very few cravings to eat when you're not hungry. How can this be? Well, remember that when you crave to eat when you're not hungry, it is for psychological reasons. If you resist the urge to eat, you will think more about the food (psychological deprivation). The more you resist urges to eat when you're not hungry, the stronger the association between whatever the psychological need and food.

For example, maybe you crave sweets when you feel lonely. If you resist eating sweets simply because you know you're not hungry, you will continue to think about the candy until the craving becomes so strong that you can't control yourself any longer and you will overeat on sweets. Now every time you feel lonely, you will do the same thing — resist. Each time you do this, your psychological deprivation is getting stronger. In fact, you may have established a rule that says, "I must never eat when I'm feeling lonely." That increases the likelihood that you will crave eating when you're lonely. Loneliness and sweets will be paired in your brain.

If, instead, you eat whenever you feel like eating, several things happen:

1) your craving is satisfied as quickly as possible; 2) since your craving is satisfied, the thoughts of food cease; 3) if there are no longer any thoughts of food, food can't be paired with your feelings of loneliness; 4) you're left now only with a clear feeling of loneliness, which you can address in effective ways without interference from a brain trying to fight psychological deprivation; and, finally, 5) once you deal directly with your loneliness, you solve it and it no longer will be a problem for you. Now the original trigger of your food craving, loneliness, has disappeared and can't trigger any more cravings in the future.

So, anyway you look at it, when it comes to food, rules have no place in your life. They will only serve to give you problems with anxiety, anger, fear, loss of control over food, and being overweight. For 20 years I've asked people to find a good reason to have rules with food. No one has ever been able to find one. Life, especially your relationship with food, is simpler and more enjoyable when you don't have rules to get in your way. If you study a naturally thin person, you'll find no food rules in her mind. So, if you want to be more like naturally thin people, start by throwing away your food rules.

Chapter 7 Tidbits

- Rules about food are made to be broken and will be broken.

- Rules about food lead to feelings of guilt, anger, and anxiety that in turn lead to failure.

- Rules about food lead to psychological deprivation, which makes the brain focus more on the food being resisted and, ultimately, leads to loss of control with that food.

- You can still have nutritional goals and desires, and strive to be better, without handicapping yourself with food rules.

- Letting go of your food rules puts you on the road to success with weight and makes your life more pleasant all the way around.

- Eating what you want, even when you're not hungry, decreases the cravings to eat when you're not hungry. That is, if you eat what you want whenever you want it, you will find you get very few cravings to eat when you're not hungry.

My "Mind Over Fat Matters" Notes

What I want to remember:

What I want to do:

How this will enrich my life:

Chapter 8

How to Eliminate the

Obsession With Food

Now we're ready for step-by-step instructions for eliminating one of the biggest psychological barriers to successful weight management: obsession with food. We've already explored how we can become obsessed in the first place. We can become too focused on food when we put weight or eating in too central a position in our lives, when we set rules about food, and when we are psychologically deprived of the foods we like. What we want is to be content with ourselves and our lives, enjoy our daily lives, enjoy food, be active individuals, and be lean, fit, and healthy. Does it sound like too much to expect? It's not. We can have all these things and it's not even that difficult to achieve as long as we accept the Laws of Life. The Laws of Life are like the Law of Gravity. They are fact, not theory. No matter how much one tries to get around them, it simply is not possible.

What are the Laws of Life? They are:

- True happiness requires self-acceptance.

- Physical health requires regular physical activity and eating quality foods.

- Inherited physiological limitations of the body cannot be conquered. Attempts to do so result in ill health (physical and mental), loss of control, and can be fatal.

- Perfection is impossible.

- Everyone is unique.

- Patience, consistency, and compassion are virtues that lead to success.

There are many more Laws of Life, but, for our purposes, this is a good starting point. Now let's get to some specifics about how to let go of those rules that have been ruling us and causing deprivation, obsession, and loss of control.

An important skill to learn in order to be able to let go of rules and, ultimately, gain natural control over eating, is what I call "self-talk." Self-talk is simply consciously talking to oneself in a rational manner in an attempt to dispute thoughts or beliefs that are causing problems in life. Humans talk to themselves all the time, but, most of the time, we aren't aware of what we're saying to ourselves. Most of the unconscious conversations we have in our minds are based on our belief systems. In our belief systems, we may have beliefs such as "One should never trust other people"; "I will never be successful"; or "Life sucks." We can just as easily have beliefs that say, "Life is wonderful"; "Most people are trustworthy"; or "I will be successful."

Everyone has known people with both types of belief systems but we are not always aware of our own belief system. What kinds of things do you believe? From our beliefs come thoughts and evaluations about other people and events that happen to us on a daily basis. For example, if Paula believes that she is unlikable and her friend is late picking her up to go somewhere, Paula is likely to think, "She probably forgot about me. I'm not important to her. I knew she didn't like me."

On the other hand, Judy, believing herself to be likable, would think, "I wonder what happened? I'll give her a few more minutes and then I'll call her. Maybe she's just stuck in traffic." Paula assumes that her friend's tardiness has to do with Paula's worth as a person. Judy doesn't connect her friend's lateness with her self-worth at all. She understands that there can be many reasons why her friend is late and, instead, will wait to find out what the reason is before making any judgment.

When it comes to our eating and weight world, beliefs can determine our success or failure. The following is a real-life case of how beliefs can become psychological barriers to success with managing our weight:

Becky was a 23-year-old college student who came to me because she was overweight and thought that I could put her on a "perfect" diet that would make her lose weight. Becky had been on many diets before and had lost weight each time, only to regain the lost weight and add a few extra pounds to it. She was an attractive and bright young woman but came across as very insecure and passive. One of our first goals in helping Becky was to make her aware of some of her beliefs that were making her fail at losing weight and keeping it off. Some of Becky's most destructive beliefs were:

"I am ugly."

"I can't do anything right."

"I'm dumb."

"I have no control over food."

"Nobody likes me."

"If I start to eat, I can't stop."

"Other people are better than me."

"If I don't follow my diet perfectly, it means I'm a failure."

Becky didn't have a chance with this type of thinking, but first I had to show her how her thoughts — not her — were keeping her from being successful, and how her beliefs had to go if she were to succeed with her weight. The second step was to show Becky how to change her beliefs to ones that would help instead of hurt her. The third step was for Becky to apply what she had learned and experience for herself that she could be successful with a new outlook about life, herself, and food.

Before we can get rid of beliefs and thoughts that are barriers to success, we have to become aware of what the thoughts are that we are repeating, unconsciously, dozens of time per day.

If you recall, rules make us feel anxious, uneasy, or just plain uncomfortable. Whenever you are feeling uncomfortable — even if you can't define the feeling itself as being anxiety or guilt or anger, for example — stop, clear your mind, and ask yourself, "What am I saying to myself right now about this situation?" Perhaps you walk into your apartment late at night and immediately feel uneasy. Stop and clear your mind. Ask, "What am I saying to myself right now?" Maybe you're saying, "I always end up wanting to eat when I get home late. I can't do that! What if I can't stop myself? There's chocolate cake in the refrigerator but I am not supposed to have it. No, no, no. I can't have it." Don't worry about what the particular thoughts say at this time. Just allow yourself to explore the dialogue that goes on within you as you go about your day.

Discovering what you say to yourself as you go about your life will be quite revealing. You won't believe the kinds of thoughts you think. The more you practice this technique, the better you will become at knowing what particular thoughts are getting in your way at any given time. You will notice patterns in your thinking. For example, your destructive thoughts may usually have to do with your expecting yourself to behave perfectly —always. Maybe you do a lot of name calling, "I'm such an idiot. What a fool I am. What a stupid thing to do." Your thoughts are valuable tools to conquering psychological barriers.

Your brain, if you recall, can be either your friend or foe. In this case, you're trying to teach your brain to stop resisting and to start helping. The quickest way to make positive changes in your thinking is to keep a journal of your dysfunctional thoughts. Get in the habit of carrying the journal around. Whenever uncomfortable feelings arise, stop to ask what the thoughts are and write them down. You'll be amazed at what you write.

The next step toward eliminating dysfunctional thoughts is to learn to dispute them. First, you have to find what's illogical or destructive in those thoughts — in what way are the thoughts hurting you instead of helping you to reach your goals? Once you have figured this out, you explain to your brain why its thinking is wrong. Yes, you actually talk to yourself — out loud, at first, unless you're in a situation where you might be thought to have gone off your rocker. Why out loud? Because your brain is used to being able to think about a lot of things at once and can easily stray. When you talk out loud, you have more focus. Actually, in the beginning, writing down the logical perspectives right after the dysfunctional thoughts is extremely helpful. When you write, the brain is forced to pay more attention.

The following is a sample journal entry from a former patient:

Situation: I was attending a party at a friend's house. I was on a diet. My friend served my favorite treat — brownies.

Illogical thoughts: "Look at those great brownies. Judy makes the best brownies ever. I can't have any. I have to lose this weight so I can't even have a bite. I want some so badly but I can't have any, I can't, I can't."

Disputing thoughts: "Yes, Judy does make wonderful brownies. There's no rule that says I can't have any. It's important that I focus more on getting rid of my rules rather than my perfectly sticking to a diet so that I will no longer lose control of my eating. If I keep telling myself I can't have the brownies when I want them, I'll psychologically deprive myself more until I won't be able to control myself and will eat more brownies than if I let myself eat some right now. So, do you really want some brownies? Okay, let's get ourselves some brownies and sit down to thoroughly enjoy them."

You won't have to keep a journal forever. The journal will simply help eliminate rules and dysfunctional thinking as quickly as possible. Before long, it will be simple to catch illogical thinking while it's happening and the thoughts can quickly be disputed. When disputing, you remind yourself of your priorities and goals, and point out to your brain the type of thinking that's going to insure that your goals will be reached. The primary goal is to live life to the fullest while feeling peaceful and happy, and being the fittest person you can be.

There are two times when humans tend to eat. We eat when we're hungry and, at times, simply for pleasure. Eating for pleasure when we're not hungry isn't abnormal. The only type of eating that is abnormal is compulsive eating. When we previously discussed compulsive eating, we saw that there is no pleasure in compulsive eating. There are certain foods that we tend to eat when we're not hungry, when we are simply looking for the pleasure of eating. These include such things as sweets and snack foods. It's also true that we rarely eat such things as celery, squash, salads, and prunes when we're not hungry (funny how these foods tend to be ones in the Fruit/Vegetable Group). What does this mean?

To me, it means that it's normal to sometimes eat when we're not hungry for the sheer psychological pleasure of it. We need pleasure in our lives for balance. If food was only supposed to be eaten when we're hungry, foods like candy bars and ice cream wouldn't exist. It's no accident that desserts are eaten at the end of a meal. We're not hungry by then. It just feels good to taste the goodies.

Think of your favorite goody. Now think of something you like, but that is just a sensible, but tasty, thing to eat, like broccoli casserole (if you like broccoli; if you don't, substitute something you like). Which food gives that giddy, childish feeling? I rest my case. So let's agree that eating only for pleasure is a normal thing. Let's also agree that it is important to our general happiness and we shouldn't deprive ourselves of it. Now we can throw out the rule that says, "I must never eat unless I'm hungry."

Now you might be thinking, "Yes, sounds good, but if I eat whenever I just want to, I'll eat junk all the time, never stop, and I'm back to being fat. This doesn't sound like a good way to lose weight and keep it off." I'm glad you're thinking and questioning what I say, but let's look at what is illogical in your assumptions. This will be a good example of being aware of your thoughts, questioning their logic, and disputing them.

The thought is: "If I eat whenever I just want to, I'll eat junk all the time, never stop, and I'm back to being fat."

What is illogical about this statement is this: You're assuming with the statement that nothing else is being done to eliminate the problems with weight and eating. On the contrary, at this point, you are working on your movement levels; you're eating more nutritious and less fattening foods at meal times; you're getting to know your psychological barriers; you're understanding how your brain works; and you are working on having the right priorities. In addition, you have learned that several things happen when you let go of rules: your psychological deprivation disappears; you lose your obsession with food and the uncontrollable cravings that result; you gain natural control over food (your body tells you what, when, and how much to eat and all is at normal levels); and you lose weight.

So, now the occasions when you want to eat something when you're not hungry will be few and far between. And on those rare occasions when you eat what you want, you will be satisfied with a modest amount and go on with your life without guilt or anxiety. It's like stopping to smell a fragrant flower. You smell it, enjoy it, and move on. So what is there really to worry about? The sooner you start letting go of rules and freeing yourself, the sooner all the problems with weight and eating will be a thing of the past. Know one thing for sure: if you keep doing what you've always done, you'll get what you've always gotten.

I've just demonstrated how to dispute a dysfunctional thought with self-talk. The more it's done, the sooner the old thoughts will go away and the logical thoughts will become a natural part of your thinking.

How can you make the transition from resisting eating when you simply want something, to eating when you want to eat, without freaking out? Take the following steps.

1) When you want to eat something, pay attention to how you are feeling. If you are feeling uncomfortable in any way — be it anxiety, fear, irritability, or tension — stop to do some self-talk.

2) Ask yourself what you have been saying to yourself about eating the desired food, and what rule may be behind it all. Perhaps you want to eat some candy after lunch and you have a rule that says, "I can't have sweets after a meal." Maybe you are also saying, "If I eat the candy, I'll be ruining my diet and everything will be messed up. If I eat the candy, I won't be able to stop and I'll get fat."

3) Now, look closely at the thoughts about eating and dispute them.

4) Remind yourself of why rules have been a problem in your life.

5) Consider your priorities and list them in order of importance.

6) Emphasize that aside from maintaining a good quality of life, you also want to become leaner and fitter, but that you want to achieve these through effective and permanent ways this time.

7) Tell yourself to take a deep breath and relax. Repeat, "There are no rules. I can have whatever I want, whenever I want it. The more I relax and eat what I want when I want it, the less I will eat in the long run."

8) Remind yourself that as you let go of rules and allow yourself to eat what you want, your eating will lessen.

9) Guide yourself by saying, "Since there are no rules, I can have some _____ (fill in the blank) now, if I want it. I can have it later, or I can choose to not have it at all until I desire it at a later point. Which do I choose? There are no rules, so if I choose not to have it now, I can change my mind at any time — even five minutes from now."

10) If you decide you want the food now, calmly take a normal portion and savor the food, reminding yourself along the way of why you are doing the right thing.

11) Once you have finished the portion you served yourself, ask, "Would I like some more?" Be careful to watch for any tension building up and dispute the thoughts that are causing the tension. Remind yourself again that you can have this food whenever you want, so you don't have to eat it now and decide. If you decide not to eat it now, emphasize that you can change your mind whenever you want and go on. If you choose to eat more, follow the previous steps again.

As you continue to guide yourself through this process, you will find yourself less and less focused on food and more focused on other things in life. Food will again be in its proper place in life. Food is a wonderful thing and is to be enjoyed. When you want it, eat it, savor it, take pleasure in it, and then go on to the next wonderful thing. You will always be coming back to enjoy food again. There are few things we do in life more often than eat. It would be sad to turn something that we do so frequently into a stressful event.

Chapter 8 Tidbits

- Use self-talk to become aware of the dysfunctional thinking that leads to your loss of control with eating.

- Dispute any illogical thoughts that are getting in the way of your weight goals. Use a journal to counteract your psychological barriers and permanently eliminate them.

- Work on letting go of food rules. Allow yourself to eat whatever you want, whenever you want it. If you want something, go for the best and eat it as soon as possible, then relax and enjoy. It will lead to eating less.

- If there are no rules, it means that you don't have to eat if you don't want to; so if you don't want a particular food right then, remember you can change your mind at any time. Don't eat it until you will really enjoy it.

- If you keep doing what you've always done, you'll get what you've always gotten.

- Keep the laws of life in focus as you begin to let go of food obsessions. Remind yourself of the importance of true happiness, self-acceptance, health, uniqueness, and patience, among other things.

- Get to know your belief system and question its power to determine success or failure with weight issues in particular and life in general.

- Remember that food should be enjoyed.

My "Mind Over Fat Matters" Notes

What I want to remember:

What I want to do:

How this will enrich my life:

Chapter 9

Improving the Quality

of What You Eat

Now that you have rediscovered natural control over eating, you have the freedom to choose to improve the quality of the food you eat. Before this point, the psychological barriers of rules, psychological deprivation, and compulsive eating thwarted your good intentions time and time again. You no longer "have to" change the quality of your eating, but rather, you can choose to change the quality of your eating. You no longer have to be perfect at achieving quality nutrition. Now, you can take steps that are tailored to your individual nature. There are no longer any deadlines for achieving better nutrition; you simply look to a lifetime of improvement. What a relief!

Good nutrition is important in preventing compulsive eating. Some compulsive eating is due to physiological factors rather than psychological ones. Sometimes your body is giving signals that it needs something in particular, but, because of all the psychological barriers you have set up, you misinterpret the signals. You may interpret your body's signal to eat as inappropriate and resist it; you may get in the way by deciding for the body what it should have and give it the wrong thing; or, after having resisted, you finally break down and gorge on just the foods you've had rules about (sweets or starches, usually). Your body may have just needed some protein but you gave it sweets, so it continues to make demands that continue to be misheard and the cycle continues. By making sure the body gets what it needs, compulsive eating for physiological reasons can easily be eliminated.

There are some simple techniques for achieving better nutrition and now is the time to learn them. You can pick and choose from any of the following methods, remembering that perfection is not expected. As with learning any new skill, practice makes better (rather than perfect), and reinforcing your efforts and successes speeds up the learning process.

A few words about self-reinforcement: There are two types of self-reinforcement that are important in acquiring new skills. The first, we might call "praise." Praise involves self-talk. Verbally giving yourself a "pat on the back" and pointing out what you've been doing well goes a long way with succeeding at many things in life. Here are some examples of good self-praise: "I ate four servings of fruits and vegetables today. Good going! I'd like to try for five servings now." "I'm doing better about relaxing when I eat and I'm catching myself when I start to tighten up."

The important thing about self-praise is that you point out the positive, the signs of improvement and effort. The negative shouldn't be dwelled upon. Telling yourself that you've fallen short will only rob you of any enthusiasm to continue your work. You know when you haven't reached a goal yet, so pointing it out will only lead to resistance from your brain. It helps to think of ourselves as children. If you're trying to teach a child to tie a bow and you slap her hand and criticize every mistake, the child gets disillusioned and loses motivation to continue trying. Instead, if praised for every small successful step and for the effort, you'll have a positive, motivated child that will succeed at tying a bow. The child's brain and the adult brain are similar when it comes to how we learn and how we become motivated.

The second type of reinforcement we might call "incentives." Everyone responds to incentives as long as you find the right incentive for you. The same way that you need to understand what type of movement you enjoy so that you will do it often enough to increase your general activity level, you need to find what types of rewards motivate you. Every person likes different things, so using the same reward for everyone doesn't work. The incentives we're interested in are small ones that don't cost much in terms of money or effort. Things like movies, time alone to relax, purchasing some small token like nail polish or a magazine, making a long-distance call to an old friend — these are examples of the type of rewards to think about.

These rewards are to be used to reinforce specific small goals, such as eating a fruit or vegetable each day. The goal should be very specific. Instead of saying, "My goal will be to eat more green vegetables every day," the goal should be more like, "My goal is to eat five green vegetables this week."

Remember that if the goal sounds too big or overwhelming, it needs to be broken up into smaller goals. Perhaps the goals need to be daily goals instead of weekly goals at first.

Barbara, a creative client of mine, made a list of 20 small rewards that pleased her. On her list were things such as nail polish, watching her favorite TV show, buying a magazine, lying in her hammock for 30 minutes, and taking a bubble bath. She set goals on a daily basis and if the goal was achieved, she could choose her reward from her list. You can be as creative as you want to be with incentives.

Notice that punishments and criticisms have no place in this reward system. Punishment *unmotivates* and gets in the way of success.

Eating better quality foods is as easy as counting on one hand. There are four high-nutrition food groups: Bread/Cereal, Fruit/Vegetable, Protein, and Milk. The goal is simply to include each food group daily in your meals. A casual focus is all that is needed here. You can pay attention to what you're eating and compare it to the four food groups. Asking, "What food groups am I missing so far today?" is an effortless check.

I haven't forgotten the fifth food group — Treats. It simply is not usually one of the high-nutrition groups, although there is no reason why you can't also get plenty of nutrition from this group. When you feel like having a treat, you can consider your options and note which treats have the most nutritional value. If your options are oatmeal-raisin cookies, jellybeans, a candy bar, or ice cream, you might note that the oatmeal-raisin cookies contain items from the Bread/Cereal Group (oatmeal) and the Fruit/Vegetable Group (raisins). The candy bar may have nuts, which come from the Protein Group, and chocolate from the Milk Group. The jellybeans are the least nutritious choice as they contain only sugar and coloring, (My husband, who loves jellybeans, says that they're a vegetable because they are a type of bean). The ice cream, of course, contains ingredients from the Milk Group and it may even contain fruit or nuts. If, after considering all this, your brain won't be satisfied unless it has jellybeans, then by all means, have them. But you'll find that having a casual focus on the nutritional content of your treats will lead to frequently choosing more nutritious ones.

Nutritional experts recommend that we eat at least five servings daily from the Fruit/Vegetable Group. The contents in fruits and vegetables have great health benefits. They have fiber, loads of vitamins, and minerals that have been shown to aid in preventing many diseases, including some cancers. You don't need to get bogged down with knowing exactly what the fruit or vegetable contains and exactly what diseases it may combat. Your job is to eat and enjoy the food, and the expert — your body — will do all the work.

Simply think of one serving to be about one-half cup to a cup, or, as in the case of something like an apple or banana, choose an average-sized item. For example, there are little bananas, average-sized bananas, and large, whopper bananas. The average-sized banana would be closest to an average serving for that food item. Remember, you don't need to be exact all the time. It all averages out.

Focusing on health rather than weight loss when it comes to changing food quality leads to more success. Anytime the brain thinks of positive things rather than negative things, and adding something rather than subtracting something, the brain relaxes and cooperates. It's easier for the brain to think about adding more green vegetables than subtracting calories or an amount of food.

Think for a second. Which feels better, thinking of eating an additional fruit today, or taking something off your plate at dinner? When you focus on the positive and what you need to add, you automatically subtract something. You automatically reduce fats and calories, so you're working in the direction of getting leaner without focusing on it.

The focus on what we eat should be a relaxed and casual one. Strive to include all the food groups in your daily eating. Generally, just knowing what foods contain the most fat and fiber is enough to improve the quality of what you eat and will help you to manage your weight successfully.

What if you're a picky eater? No problem. Few can be as picky as I was earlier in my life. My mother never cooked a green vegetable. Our vegetables consisted of corn and potatoes. We ate almost exclusively chicken, beef, pork, rice, beans, corn, and potatoes. I wasn't familiar with most other foods until I became a young adult and went to college. By that time, anything I hadn't tasted, I would simply say I didn't like, particularly anything green.

How did I become a well-nourished person? I stopped saying I didn't like something. Instead, I said to myself that I hadn't yet found a form of the food that I liked. I started to search and experiment for things I liked by trying different recipes. I discovered, for example, that I didn't like cooked spinach, but I liked fresh spinach in a salad that included lots of other things that I liked. I also liked spinach in things like casseroles with cheese or rice — anything that tasted more like the other foods rather than the spinach. As long as I ate the spinach I got the nutrition. It didn't matter how I fooled my brain into eating it.

So, if you're a picky eater, stop using that as an excuse and experiment. Even if you find that you can't eat liver, no matter how you present it to your brain, there will be other things you will be able to eat, enjoy, and gain health from.

With all that said, here's to your health!

Chapter 9 Tidbits

- The quality of what you eat is extremely important in your weight-loss success. By making sure that your body gets the nutrients it needs, you keep everything functioning at top efficiency (including fat burning), and you avoid overeating.

- Improving the quality of what you eat should not be complicated. A casual focus on including all food groups daily, and knowing generally what types of foods contain the most fats and fiber, is most of what you need to know to eat more nutritiously.

- Self-talk and reinforcement are useful tools in making changes with your food quality. Any time the brain thinks of positive things rather than negative things, and of adding something rather than subtracting something, the brain relaxes and cooperates.

- If you focus on health rather than weight loss, and stop making excuses about being a picky eater, you will go a long way towards creating a leaner, healthier body.

- Practice makes better, not perfect. The goal is just to improve through practice. Perfection is an unrealistic goal and striving for it only leads to constant feelings of failure.

- If there are nutritious foods you don't like or think you don't like, try different recipes with these foods to see if there are ways that you might like them. If you still don't like them, don't worry about it. Have other foods that give you some of the same good things but continue to strive for variety.

My "Mind Over Fat Matters" Notes

What I want to remember:

What I want to do:

How this will enrich my life:

Chapter 10

"My Eyes Are Bigger Than My Stomach" Phenomenon: Dealing With Portion Control

Everyone knows that portion control is important in losing weight. Even "all-you-can-eat" diets ultimately function on the fact that eating is reduced. The problem, as we have mentioned before, is that the brain doesn't like to have things taken away. It deals better when things are added rather than subtracted. So, how do we reduce portions without our brain protesting? We simply use the same methods we've used with changing our activity level, our nutrition, and our psychological barriers, along with a few creative tips that we'll cover ahead.

If the brain always told us to eat only what we needed, no one would likely ever be overweight. If we were inactive, the brain would just tell us to eat less. If we were more active on any given day, it would have us eat more to cover the extra energy expended.

As you know, life isn't that simple. There are several factors that determine your appetite from one moment to another. Some things that affect appetite are stress, habit, what types of foods you are eating, your degree of hunger, and psychological deprivation.

Everyone responds differently to stress. In the same way that some people experience stress by getting headaches, having stomach problems, or breaking out in a rash, our individual appetites can respond differently to the same types and degrees of stress. Some people lose their appetite when they're stressed, while others feel like eating compulsively. Some people eat more when they're moderately nervous and lose their appetite when the stress is intense, like when a loved one has died or there is a divorce. Generally speaking, most people lose their appetite when their stress level is intense but there are always exceptions. Whatever your reaction to stress, it's normal for you, so accept it, don't fight it. Instead, you're here to learn how to deal with your individual tendencies in response to the stress in your life.

Habit is another factor that affects appetite and, therefore, the portions that we serve ourselves. Habits can be broken — True or False? The answer is "True," but habits are not broken easily by using cold-turkey methods. Just as with Pavlov's dog, if you usually eat under certain conditions, your brain will pair eating with that situation, and will signal you to eat whenever you are in the same circumstances.

For example, if you start eating every night while watching your favorite TV programs, you will start salivating and your stomach will start releasing gastric juices to prepare for eating. You feel it as hunger or simply as a craving for your usual TV snacks. If you try to keep yourself from eating, your brain will keep insisting that you obey its demands, making it next to impossible to deny it (at least that's how it feels to you).

Habit change has to be gradual in order to be successful and to keep it from being torturous. The more patient and creative you are, the sooner and more comfortable habit changing will be. Be assured, however, that it's simpler than most people think, because most use the "grit-your-teeth-and-bear-it" approach.

Using positive rewards for small advances with habit changing is the key to keeping motivated and feeling good about small successes. Remember to choose your rewards according to the things that work for you, things that you like or value. If you don't give a hoot about going shopping, don't use that as a reward for taking a walk instead of watching TV. Make the reinforcer fit you.

The types of foods you eat and their nutritional value also have an effect on appetite and, consequently, the amounts you eat. The reasons for this are primarily physiological. The brain's job is to keep you alive and well. If you eat poorly, your brain will attempt to get you to eat what you need. When you don't provide the body with what it needs, then you will have a tendency to eat too much of the foods you do eat.

It's also true that eating too much sugar or starchy, non-nutritive foods (like white breads, pastas, and cereals), to the exclusion of other more nutritious food groups, can play havoc with insulin levels in your body, which have a direct effect on hunger and appetite.

Having little fiber in your diet also contributes to overeating. Fiber is filling. A high-fiber diet is generally a lower-calorie diet than one that is lacking in fiber. These are other reasons why consuming a balance of all of the major food groups is so important. The better fed you are, the less you will overeat.

Many people try to ignore hunger when they're trying to lose weight. It's all in an attempt to consume less, but what they usually don't know is that they are setting themselves up to eat more in the long run. Ignoring hunger only adds to your psychological deprivation and slows down metabolism, so you end up with a double whammy. You put yourself in a situation where you're going to eat more compulsively and store fat more readily.

It's wise to catch hunger early. Feed the body as soon as it starts to give signals that it needs to be fed. A small amount of hunger requires smaller amounts of food for satisfaction. Big amounts of hunger require big amounts of food to make you feel satisfied and, if you have large amounts of psychological deprivation, you may not feel satisfied even after getting full. So, if you're hungry, eat!

Finally, there is psychological deprivation. We've said a lot about this subject already. Suffice it to say that the more psychologically deprived you are because of food rules, the larger the portions you'll eat. When you have an opportunity to eat, your brain will respond by thinking something like: *I'm going to eat as much as I can right now that I have the opportunity, because I don't know when I'll be fed again.* If you're not psychologically deprived, you know that you can eat whenever you want, so there's no need to stuff yourself now.

A good example of how food rules can affect portion control is when you have rules that say something like this: "I must never have seconds. I must always have smaller-than-average portions. I must always eat less than everybody else." You've learned enough in this book now to get a sense of what the brain will think and feel when being reminded of these rules. It will feel deprived and will feel like resisting — something like: *This may be the last time I get to eat _____ so I want more.* The brain definitely will not be satisfied with the portion that you are demanding it gets. When you feel this way, the likelihood is that sooner or later, you will have more than you had planned — your portions will be bigger rather than smaller. Instead, if you don't have a rule about portions, you won't be psychologically deprived. You know you can have whatever you want whenever you want it, so its value will be more realistic and the urge to eat will be lessened; therefore, portions will be smaller.

How fast you eat can also have a significant impact on the size of the portions that you end up eating at any meal. The brain needs some time to realize that it is full or feels satisfied. When you eat too fast, you end up eating larger portions of food, only to feel the frustration later that you could have done with less. Everyone has experienced this before (usually when they've allowed themselves to get too hungry), but some people tend to eat fast all the time. By slowing down your eating, you are better able to savor your food so that the brain gets as many signals as possible, and will be better able to tell when it has gotten all that it needs.

Slowing down eating is simple. First, focus on your breathing. Eat with your mouth closed, taking deep, relaxing breaths while you eat. Don't put any more food into your mouth until you have completely swallowed the previous bite, and focus on slowing down. While you are eating, focus on all the qualities of the food, such as its color, texture, and taste. It helps even to talk to yourself about what's good about the meal: "Boy, this is a good salad. I love all the beautiful colors in it and this cheese really brings out the tanginess of the orange slices." It even helps to pay attention to how you are sitting, making sure that you are in a comfortable position and definitely not standing while you're eating. If you're one of those people that eats fast all the time, it will take some practice but, before long, you'll be eating more slowly, enjoying it more, and eating smaller portions.

Chapter 10 Tidbits

Portion control can best be achieved by following these guidelines:

- Be conscious of your stress level and try to keep it under control. Whatever your reaction to stress, it's normal for you so don't fight it. You can counteract stress if you learn to be active, think positively, keep your priorities straight, don't spread yourself too thin, and enjoy relaxing pastimes.

- Be aware of habits that are getting in the way of your weight management. Set small progressive goals toward eliminating these habits. Use positive reinforcement as an incentive for change and be patient with yourself. If you backtrack, take it in stride and get back on the gradual track of improvement.

- Work at increasing the quality, including the amount of fiber, of what you eat. Use your already-learned methods of reinforcement and goal setting. Be willing to experiment with foods and recipes in order to increase quality and enjoyment of eating.

- Avoid getting extremely hungry. It's best to respond to hunger as soon as possible and to eat what you really want. Serve yourself average portions of food, despite the hunger level, while telling yourself, "I'll give myself an average portion of this food and savor it. Afterwards, and only afterwards, I will decide if I want more. If I want more, I will again serve myself average portions until my body tells me it doesn't want anymore. If I decide to stop, I know that I can eat again — there are no rules." By using self-talk, before you know it, you will naturally desire average portions and usually feel satisfied after just one meal of average portions.

- Watch out for rule-setting to avoid psychologically depriving yourself. If you notice any rules lurking around, focus on letting them go by relaxing and allowing yourself to have what you want through the methods learned in Chapter 8.

- Slow down. By slowing down your eating, you are better able to savor your food so that the brain gets as many signals as possible telling it when it has gotten all that it needs.

My "Mind Over Fat Matters" Notes

What I want to remember:

What I want to do:

How this will enrich my life:

Chapter 11

M-M-M-M Good: Savoring

Many people believe that the more they focus on food, the less they will eat. However, when you're psychologically deprived, your focus on food is of a compulsive nature. You're trying to avoid food against the needs of your body. As a result, you become more obsessed than focused. When you focus on food in a positive way, however, you can better appreciate it, and that leads to eating more normally and to more success with managing your weight.

When you savor food, you use all of the body's senses — including touch, smell, sight, and sound — in order to get the most pleasure out of each bite of food. Your goal with food should be to eat what you want and need, get pleasure out of it, feel satisfaction, and then go on to something else in life. In order to be able to do this, you need to savor your food.

Everyone is born with the ability to savor food. Just watch a baby as it suckles from its mother's breast to watch savoring in action. Through strict dieting and buying into many of the diet-crazy messages you hear around you today, you can become out of touch with your ability to savor food. You may hear that food is bad, or that you should feel guilty if you eat the "wrong" things. One day you learn that one food is good for you and that another is bad, and the next day you may hear the opposite. It's no wonder Americans are frustrated when it comes to something as natural and simple as eating!

The brain feels satiation by getting signals from your senses. You smell the wonderful aromas of a plateful of turkey, cranberries, and mashed pota-

71

toes and gravy from Thanksgiving dinner. You taste the tangy sweetness of Key lime pie. You feel the crunchiness of the fresh, crisp potato chips that accompany your mouth-watering hotdog, which you hear pop as you dig your teeth into it. Your body goes through many chemical reactions when you eat and they all contribute to the resulting feeling of satiation. When you're satiated your brain says, "That was good, but I've had enough. I'm done for now."

Our modern lifestyles aren't conducive to savoring our meals. We're often rushed, rarely eat together as a family, and food is often over-processed and unappetizing. It's time to get back to our roots and start savoring food again. It's one of the most effective ways of feeling satisfied quickly and having less urges to overeat.

Relearning to savor can be fun. First, serve colorful foods. The brain responds positively to a variety of colors on a plate. An over-processed, grayish burger on a white bun with dull, yellow, French fries isn't as exciting to the brain as a plate sprinkled with greens, reds, yellows, oranges, and golden-browns from a salad of dark green lettuce, red and yellow peppers, bright orange carrots, orange slices, lightly broiled chicken, and whole grain bread or pasta. Even the dessert can be colorful.

Don't forget the plate itself. I often encourage my patients to find colorful or fun plates, cups and glasses for their meals. If they don't have any, I tell them to go buy some. Remember how much fun it was as a kid to eat from your favorite bowls, plates, and utensils? We loved having our favorite cartoon characters accompany us at mealtime. It's no different now. You can even have cartoon characters again if it feels good to you.

The second important step in relearning to savor food is to eat in a relaxing environment. This means sitting down, choosing a favorite spot (even if it's not a typical eating place), swallowing each bite before taking another, and preventing distractions (such as TV, talking on the phone, and working). How and where you eat is almost as important as what you eat.

Third, you need to focus on using your senses while you eat. In the beginning you may have to consciously use self-talk to help yourself attend to the smells, taste, sight, and texture of the food. Before long the brain will automatically be saying things like, "Wow, this sure looks appetizing. Everything looks so fresh and I love the colors I put together in this salad. I think I'll have some of those fresh peaches for dessert. Putting some cherries and whipped cream on top sounds good, too." The brain will no longer be distracted with other unrelated and stressful matters. It now has the freedom to think about what's right in front of it — food.

A bit more about tasting: You need to taste your food like a connoisseur savors wine. The connoisseur carefully looks at the visual qualities of the wine, and then takes a nice, big mouthful, which is slowly swished throughout the mouth as he or she contemplates the different flavors present in the wine. So it should be with food. You don't have to look as silly as the wine connoisseur, and you certainly don't want to spit your food back out, but, it is important to take a large enough bite to be able to capture the essence of the food and get the full enjoyment.

This concept is especially important with foods that come in small bits, such as nuts, jellybeans, and popcorn. Don't try to control the amount of these foods by putting tiny bits in your mouth at a time. Putting one peanut in your mouth when you desire to eat peanuts is only going to frustrate your brain. Its reaction to miniscule amounts is likely to be to push you to have another and another and another, until you find that you've eaten the whole bowl or package and feel overstuffed with peanuts. Instead, take a nice mouthful of peanuts at a time and slowly savor it. Pretend you're a connoisseur of peanuts. The brain will get a nice, big, burst of signals at one time, and won't feel frantic as it would if you were giving it microscopic bits. You'll find, in the end, you'll consume fewer peanuts.

Relearning to savor food is probably one of the easiest and most enjoyable things to have to do in managing your weight. Your brain will be giddy over it.

Chapter 11 Tidbits

- Savoring food means using the body's senses (touch, smell, sight, and sound) to get the most pleasure out of each bite that you eat.

- Savoring food is second nature. Even if you've forgotten how to do it, it can easily be relearned.

- Savoring food provides signals to the brain, informing it of when your needs are met. This makes you feel satisfied with less food.

- You can better savor what you eat by serving colorful foods, using colorful plates, eating in a relaxing environment, preventing distractions, using self-talk, swallowing thoroughly before taking another bite — in short, eating like a connoisseur.

My "Mind Over Fat Matters" Notes

What I want to remember:

What I want to do:

How this will enrich my life:

Chapter 12

Dealing With Snack Foods

Snacks foods are very much a part of our American lifestyle. If you have any doubt, take a walk through a supermarket and note the wide variety of snacking delights available. The list is endless, but just to name a few, we have dozens of different types of chips, pretzels, cookies, ice cream, candies, popcorn, candy bars, sodas, nuts, crackers, and chocolates from which to choose. Let's face it — they're good. Everyone likes at least one category of these snack foods.

Snack foods per se aren't bad. Many of these goodies can provide some good things — ice cream has calcium, popcorn is high in fiber, and oatmeal cookies have fiber and iron, among other things. Snack foods become a problem only when we consume too much of them or eat them as a substitute for a nutritional meal. When snack foods replace more nutritious foods, the excess snack food calories are turned into excess stored fat. Or, we create destructive habits of eating snack foods while doing things like watching TV, working, reading, or while in bed.

Expecting the average person to stay away from snack foods is unrealistic. As we've already learned, setting rules leads to the brain becoming psychologically deprived and wanting more of the "taboo" food. More importantly, if we ask someone what his or her favorite food is, most often it's some type of snack food. Life isn't much fun if you can't eat your favorite foods, and trying to stay away from your "warm fuzzies" just makes it difficult to control yourself when you do eat them.

The mistakes most people make when dealing with snack foods include: 1) eating in situations where you can't thoroughly savor the food; 2) eating when you're not relaxed; 3) eating too fast; 4) trying to control snack eating by putting only tiny bits of the tasty treats in your mouth at a time; 5) not thoroughly swallowing before taking the next bite; and 6) not focusing enough on the taste of the food; and 7) feeling guilt about eating the treats.

Some environments just aren't conducive to enjoying eating. In our hectic lifestyles many places are too stressful, too noisy, or too busy for good savoring. At such times, it is best to look for gentler surroundings or, if at all possible and comfortable, postpone eating until you can eat calmly and have a good time with it.

There are situations, of course, where you're either too hungry, or maybe you're in the process of working on letting go of rules, so it's important to eat as soon as your brain tells you, but, otherwise, do yourself a favor and wait. Personally, I'd rather forgo eating a treat in the car in favor of eating it when I get home and get in my hammock surrounded by flowers and a beautiful lake. There I can focus on every spoonful of my toffee ice cream.

The same concept applies to when you feel tense or stressed. It may feel like a good idea to eat that candy bar at your desk while at work, perhaps just after you've been told of a deadline you think is next to impossible, but it's not. In reality, it's smarter to take a deep breath and think of how to relax so you can enjoy the chocolatey goodness. If you don't, you run the risk of feeling like eating a second candy bar simply because, at that moment, the stress is more in control of you than you are.

By now, you know the dangers of eating too fast. You don't enjoy your food and you tend to overeat when you scarf it down. Snack foods are treats and treats are meant for pleasure, so take pleasure in eating those goodies and you'll eat less of them. For example, before I sat down to finish this chapter, I relaxed in a comfortable spot and ate a small bowl of taco chips (a favorite of mine) and a glass of orange juice. I added the orange juice to increase the nutritional content of my snack. I had already intended to work on this chapter that afternoon, but I decided that since I wanted to have some chips and a drink, I would do it before sitting down to write. After all, I knew I wouldn't get as much pleasure if I ate them while I was working. I also knew that I would eat more chips and I would eat them faster if I tried to work at the same time. It's good to learn from experience.

Since savoring and satiation require that the brain receive enough messages about the food you're eating, it stands to reason that you need to take bites big enough to provide these messages and that you swallow each bite before taking the next one. Let's be thankful that the goal here is more rather than less. The behavior change you need to make is one of addition rather than subtraction. You don't have to try to put less food in your mouth or take tinier bites. The brain is a lot more cooperative when you're not taking something away from it.

Since many people feel that snack foods are "bad" foods, the tendency is to feel guilty when you eat them. How often do you hear yourself (or someone else) make excuses if you're seen eating snack foods? "Oh, this is all I've gotten to eat all day"; "I know I shouldn't be eating this"; or, "I'm getting back on my diet on Monday." What is there to feel guilty about? Eat, drink and be merry. As a matter of fact, be a model of how to enjoy food to those around you. Practice saying, "Would you like some?" "This is simply wonderful." "I love chocolate." Or, better yet, don't say anything. Just enjoy.

When a person is relaxed they naturally eat more slowly, savor better, eat less, and enjoy more. If all this sounds indulgent, it is. You should not be concerned with being too indulgent when it comes to your health and physiology. Remember to leave eating, in general, to your brain and body. They are the experts, and as long as you don't get in the way, the choices they make, more often than not, will be the right ones.

Chapter 12 Tidbits

- Snack foods are not bad foods. They give us pleasure and some can also provide good nutrients.

- When selecting snack foods, think both of what you really want and how to also make that snack more nutritious.

- Take the time to relax, savor, eat slowly, and choose a comfortable environment when having your treats.

- Above all, throw guilt out the window and embrace the pleasure of eating.

My "Mind Over Fat Matters" Notes

What I want to remember:

What I want to do:

How this will enrich my life:

Chapter 13

Eating Out and Drinking

Two effective ways to gain weight gradually and unconsciously are to add frequent eating out and drinking to your normal eating lifestyle. When I speak of drinking, I'm talking primarily about drinking anything with calories in it, such as non-diet sodas, shakes, juices, and alcoholic drinks. Alcoholic drinks are double-edged swords, but we'll get to that later.

Eating out and drinking frequently will not put fat on quickly — like compulsive eating might — but put on weight, they will. It will seem like the weight is creeping up from nowhere. It's easy to think that a drink has little or no calories (it goes down so smoothly), and eating out just seems like you're just having another meal — you had to eat lunch anyway, you just did it in a restaurant. So how did you suddenly gain 10 extra pounds? It's easy. Let's take a look.

One of the first things to realize is that restaurants are businesses. They want you to keep coming back. You wouldn't go back to a restaurant if the food doesn't taste good, so restaurants try very hard to make their food tasty. The ingredients that add the most taste to food are fat, sugar, salt, and other spices. Typically, the lower the quality of the food served in a restaurant, the more fat, sugar, and salt are added to the food to make it palatable. That's because the lower the quality of the food, the less pleasurable taste it is likely to have.

Restaurant owners aren't going to fool around much with other spices because of added cost, and they're not going to be concerned with your health or weight. Remember, profit is the concern here. If it's an expensive restaurant, it doesn't mean the food is going to be less fattening. It may mean that the food (depending on what you choose) is more nutritious because of better quality foods, but it may still be loaded with fat from rich butters, oils, and sauces.

Although sugars and salts are not as calorie-laden as fats, they have an effect on the amount of food that you eat. Sugar affects insulin levels in your body and insulin levels are connected to hunger levels. Salt has been a favorite spice of humans for centuries and it was once used as currency (that's pretty darn valuable). People love it and we consume tons of it — much more than we need.

The interesting thing about sugar and salt is that the more of them you use in your daily eating, the less you're able to detect or taste the natural sugars and salt already present in foods. Conversely, the less of them you eat, the better able you are to taste and savor the natural salt and sugars in your meals and, therefore, be satisfied with less of them. Besides, natural forms of sugars and salts are going to be better for you anyway. Finally, this isn't understood quite well yet, but high sugar and salt diets seem to have some connection to food cravings (cravings for sugar and salt). Logically, when your cravings to eat are greater, you consume more calories and are more likely to get fatter.

Now, I'm not trying to say that you should never go out to eat. After all, eating out is fun and it tastes good. Chronic dieters have many myths about eating out. Many believe that the way to control their eating when dining out is by ordering only salads, always skipping dessert, ordering food as plain as possible, or (above all) avoiding favorite foods. Nothing could be further from the truth. As a matter of fact, using these methods will ultimately lead to breaking all the rules.

Eating out in these ways is no fun, either. Unless you like salads a whole lot, forget about always eating salads. If you always skip dessert, you're going to miss out on some fantastic treats. No, as we've discussed before, eating needs to be enjoyable, and psychologically depriving yourself only leads to loss of control of eating. If you don't care much about eating out, then it's simple. Cut it down to only those times when there is no other choice. However, if you're like most other Americans and like it considerably, there are some simple steps you can take toward still having the pleasures of eating out but reducing its effect on your weight. You can choose all or any of the following pointers:

- Take note of how often you eat out each week and gradually reduce the number of times by one less each week. For example, if you tend to eat out five times per week, set the goal at four times, then three, then two, and so forth. If reducing by one time each week seems too fast, then stretch it out. What is important is that you gradually and consistently eat out less often than you did before.

- When you do eat out, think about what you are going to order with respect to its nutritional, caloric, fat, sugar, and salt contents. Don't get too uptight about it, though. Keep a positive and relaxed attitude. Then think about how you can reduce the calorie content and increase the nutrition of what you are ordering. For example, if you're thinking of ordering your usual double hamburger, you can consider a single patty, no mayo, double tomato, no pickles (they're high in salt), or chicken instead of a burger (or all of the above, for that matter). If you have control over how something is cooked, take control. Order items broiled instead of fried, or ask that half the oil or butter be used.

- Once your food arrives, take a minute to look it over. Think about where most of the nutrition and fat are located on your plate. Consider if there are ways you can still increase fiber and nutrition — and lower sugars, salts, calories, fats, or quantity — without depriving yourself.

I remember using this method just recently with some airline food. I was served a chicken dish with veggies and rice, salad, bread and butter, and a cookie. I considered the fact that, while on vacation, the quality of nutrition I had gotten was poor, at best. I decided that I would try to get the most nutrition and least fat from my airline meal as I could. I decided to increase my fiber by eating the salad and veggies. I reduced fat content by passing up the butter and cookie, and by dipping my salad in the dressing rather than pouring it on. I didn't pass up the bread because it's my favorite food and I felt that I would feel too psychologically deprived if I didn't eat it. I made sure I ate the chicken because I knew my protein intake that day was deficient. Finally, I ordered some orange juice as a good source of Vitamin C and for the sweet taste. My feeling of satisfaction at the end of the meal told me I had made the right decisions.

- Focus on relaxing and eating slowly. There are a lot more fun things about eating out than just eating. Pay attention to the atmosphere and the company. Take it all in.

- Consider the fact that you don't have to eat everything on your plate. It will feel better to be pleasantly full rather than stuffed. As a matter of fact, if the food is good, you could get two meals for the price of one by taking some home and having it the next day for lunch. Think of how much you'll like it when you look in the fridge tomorrow to find some more of that delicious vegetable lasagna.

We all know how alcohol can loosen up our behavior. It can make you feel less inhibited, giving you the courage to talk to someone you find fiercely attractive, or make you laugh without regard to a less-than-funny joke. In the same way, it disinhibits your eating in a number of ways. It can make you lose touch with signals that your body has had enough food. By the end of the night, not only have you consumed a lot of extra calories from the alcohol you drank, but the alcohol also made you eat more than you would have if you hadn't numbed yourself with the drinking.

Social drinking isn't bad in and of itself. However, if you wish to manage your weight effectively, drinking caloric drinks, in general, and drinking alcohol, in particular, is something to consider as important. Again, don't set rules. Rules are only meant to be broken. The goal is to learn what's getting in the way of managing your weight effectively and getting those things out of your way.

If you want to lessen the effect of alcohol on your eating, there are some simple steps you can take. First, try to do your drinking before or — better yet — after the meal, rather than with the meal. If you drink before the meal, try to allow enough time for the alcohol's effects to have passed before ordering your meal. There are no hard-and-fast rules here. With time, you will learn what works for you.

Second, limit the number of alcoholic drinks or space them out (my best friend does this) by having a glass of water between each drink. And third, decide whether you would rather drink or eat your extra calories, then choose either the drink or some other tasty treat (dessert, butter on your bread, cheese on your potato, etc.). Think about which is easier to give up and which would be most pleasant to have.

Here is an important side note. There is also no rule that says you have to drink alcohol. If it's not that big a deal to you and you find that you are only doing it to be sociable, skip it. Your body doesn't need alcohol, there is little nutrition in it, and you can use the calories in a more pleasurable and effective way. *It's okay not to drink at all.* If you do drink, remember the laws against drinking and driving and remember to be responsible.

A dieter's approach to eating out leads to psychological deprivation, stress, fear, and loss of control, not to mention, little or no enjoyment. A drunken brain can't help with much, least of all, trying to lose weight. The brain needs to be allowed to be free to enjoy the activity of eating out without feeling deprived. At the same time, the brain can playfully be coaxed into keeping control of your food and drink intake by presenting many and varied choices for it to make.

Chapter 13 Tidbits

- Focus on quality, know what you want to eat, and plan around that.

- Think of what you can sacrifice without feeling deprived. Remind yourself that you can take leftover food with you, so you don't have to eat everything on your plate.

- Limit caloric drinks, especially alcoholic drinks, or forgo drinking them altogether.

- Gradually reduce the frequency of eating out.

My "Mind Over Fat Matters" Notes

What I want to remember:

What I want to do:

How this will enrich my life:

Chapter 14

In the Closet:

Dealing With Compulsive Eating

Compulsive eating is not a rare thing these days, nor is there anything to be ashamed of if you have done it. It is not a sign of weakness, as many people think. If you compulsively eat, there is a logical reason for it, and the logical thing to do is to find out the cause and go about taking sensible steps toward eliminating it. So far, in discussing all the many subjects of this book, we've gone about things in a rational, logical, and positive manner. This subject will be no different.

First, let's look at defining compulsive eating. Compulsive eating is marked by three major characteristics:

- When someone eats compulsively, she doesn't eat in a relaxed and calm fashion. On the contrary, compulsive eating is marked by such feelings as tension, anxiety, and frustration.
- When someone eats compulsively, she doesn't savor the food, but rather, eats in a rapid manner, paying little attention to what she's eating.
- When someone eats compulsively, she feels out of control of her eating. She tends to feel driven to eat, rather than feeling a simple, pleasant desire to eat.

Compulsive eating isn't that much fun. People don't eat compulsively because they want to do so. They are driven to do it. The leading cause of compulsive eating is stringent dieting. The irony is that, often times, the stringent dieter is dieting as an attempt to control her compulsive eating. The dieter responds to loss of control by restricting herself more and setting more rules about her eating. These methods, unfortunately, lead to more compulsive eating.

Again, we have a case of good intentions based on misinformation. The brain will lead a person to compulsively eat whenever it is either physiologically or psychologically deprived. In past chapters, we've discussed the importance of providing your body with good nutrition, and, at the same time, not psychologically depriving yourself of foods you like and want. The brain does marvelous things to help you survive in this world and make your life worth living. These are things worthy of appreciation. By the brain doing so much for you automatically, it allows you to take part in scores of other things that life has to offer that add to your happiness.

Your brain is your partner in life, so when something seems to be going wrong, it may actually be right. If you're depriving your body of proper nutrition, you should be thankful that your brain nudges you lightly, or not so lightly, to eat. If you are hurting yourself by psychologically depriving yourself, and you find yourself compulsively eating, it's your brain saying, "Hey, wake up. Pay attention and stop this foolishness. Things are off balance here and we need to correct it now."

Instead of resisting the signals from your brain, listen to them and use the skills you've been learning here to get back in natural control. The person who doesn't chronically deprive herself doesn't compulsively eat, because she is consistently listening to her brain and following its lead. Compulsive eating only happens when one doesn't listen to the brain and resists its natural control. This causes interference, so to speak, and the messages become garbled.

For example, your brain may be telling you to eat some fruit, but you're so psychologically deprived that you instead start obsessing with the foods that you have rules about (such as sweets and other snacks), and end up compulsively eating the cookies you had vowed not to eat. It was fruit that your body needed, but your brain was so full of other junk that you misinterpreted the messages and were afraid to listen to them. When you get rid of your psychological deprivation and provide your body with good nutrition in your daily eating, compulsive eating will become a thing of the past.

Eliminating dieting is the first step in stopping compulsive eating. By doing so, you will finally provide your body with enough calories, fiber, vitamins and minerals, and foods that contribute to your emotional well-being.

You will be in balance, both physiologically and psychologically, and your brain will have no reason to compel you to eat.

How do you eliminate dieting? Here are a few reminders:

- Get rid of rules.

- Savor food.

- Have a casual focus on food.

- Make sure all food groups are included daily.

- Learn to relax and enjoy life.

Compulsive eating isn't natural, but it's not a sign of weakness in character. Depriving yourself of food, or feeling guilt over having done so, can't solve the problem. There are logical and simple reasons for why someone may be compulsively eating and there's definitely a solution to the problem. So lighten up and take it one step at a time and, before long, you'll experience the beauty of natural control over food.

Chapter 14 Tidbits

- Compulsive eating is nothing to be ashamed of. It doesn't mean that you're weak or lack self-discipline. It does mean that you're going about things in an incorrect way and, the sooner you learn the correct way, the quicker you'll be free of eating compulsively.

- Stringent dieting is the major cause of compulsive eating. Eliminating strict dieting is the first step toward gaining natural control and never compulsively eating again.

- The reasons for compulsive eating can be physiological or psychological (usually it's both). If you deprive your body nutritionally and/or deprive it psychologically through food rules, you will set yourself up to eat compulsively.

- Getting rid of rules, savoring food, including all food groups in your daily eating, and relaxing will prevent compulsive eating.

My "Mind Over Fat Matters" Notes

What I want to remember:

What I want to do:

How this will enrich my life:

Chapter 15

Playful Exercise

In Chapter 3, we generally discussed the role of exercise in successful weight loss. You learned that looking at exercise as movement, rather than as exercise, helps the brain to think positively about the idea. It will be less likely to resist your efforts to become a more active and leaner person. We know that exercise is good for us and that it definitely helps the body burn more fat, but few people have exercise as a regular part of their lifestyle. Most people will say that they want to exercise, but they really don't "want" to exercise. That is to say, most people wish they would exercise but find the whole thought of it distasteful. That's the brain talking.

Sure, your brain knows that exercise is good for your health and would make losing weight faster and more permanent. All this is logical to the brain (it's an intellectual exercise). At the same time, though, the thought of exercise conjures up associations of discomfort, tension, failures, and other negative things. These associations have been made because of longstanding rules you've set that you "have to" or "need to," or that you "should" exercise for whatever reasons (usually that you "have to" lose weight). At this point the brain isn't thinking intellectually anymore. It's thinking emotionally and, emotionally, the brain can't stand the thought of something that's going to cause so much psychological and physical pain. The brain is a clever brain. It has all kinds of tricks up its brainy sleeve that will help you avoid such torture as exercise.

Children exercise all the time but no one calls it exercise. It's playing, or "they're just being kids." Somehow, we don't think that adults can be as active, or that they should be as active or that adults can play. Sure, children tend to have more energy than most adults and, sure, children don't have the responsibilities that we adults have, but here's the secret. Adults can play, too. Not just when it's allowed or planned, such as when we go to a football game or go on vacation, but every day of our lives. Wow, what a novel idea! "I can play?" you ask. Yes, you can play. You can play everyday, whenever you want to play, and you can play at everything and anything you do.

For example, I can think of the writing I'm doing right now as work — a chore (which I have done many times) — or I can look at it as an opportunity to play. If I play with my writing, I think things like, *Oh, good. I get to sit here awhile and just see what comes out of my mind. I get to write down whatever feels good. This is like an adventure.*

If, on the other hand, I think of writing as a chore, I'll probably avoid it at all costs. I'll figure I really need to return some phone calls first. Then my internal dialogue goes like this: *I really should go through the mail. I can't possibly write while the office is so messy.* Some days all these other priorities take all day so I conclude that, *I just never had the time to write.* If I'm able to force myself to sit down and start writing, not only will I not have any fun, but my writing reflects it. Playing at writing is so much more fun and I'm more successful with it if I play at it.

This is also true with exercise. In Chapter 3, we discussed ways of playing your way into a more active lifestyle. It helps a great deal to accept who you are and only do the forms of movement that are the most enjoyable, even if what you like is jumping out of a box over and over again. Don't concern yourself with what the movement is, as long as you take the attitude of playing and are encouraged to keep doing it as a result of that attitude.

Dieters make a lot of mistakes with exercise. A person can exercise excessively to the point where the exercise loses it appeal, or where it can actually be damaging to the body physically or psychologically (making it impossible to continue exercising).

One of my favorite clients, a perky, sweet woman of only 21 years, loved to dance. She decided to use dance as her form of movement to help her lose weight. That was a smart and creative thing to do. The problem was that she then expected to dance three hours every day without fail. Dance, instead of her love, became her chore. She was no longer treating dancing as play, now it was a job. It was so excessive that she became exhausted and couldn't keep up the pace.

A second mistake that people make with exercise is expecting to get results too fast, or setting goals that are too big. I can use myself as a good example for this one. For a couple of years, I had wanted to learn to be a jogger like my (then) boyfriend. I had asthma at the time, but I would see other people start to jog and within a week, they were able to jog a mile consistently without stopping to walk (or so I thought). Other people seemed to just glide along the jogging track with the greatest of ease and I thought I should be able to do the same. So, I would set out jogging at more of a running pace (much too fast for my fitness level at the time) and I would expect myself to finish the mile without stopping or slowing down.

I would compare myself to the other runners every step of the way. Well, of course, I couldn't finish the mile without stopping, and I didn't let myself forget that all the way home. I don't have to tell you that I quit trying before the week was up. I expected to become fit enough to run the entire mile before it was possible for my body to do so. My expectations and goals were too big. I was destined to fail with this strategy.

When I finally came to my senses, I realized that if ever I was to reach my ultimate goal of running a mile without stopping and, more importantly, continue to be active for the rest of my life, I would have to do several things. First, I would have to stop comparing myself to others; it didn't matter how long it took me to be able to run the complete mile as long as I kept trying. Second, I would have to start where I was; I was asthmatic and unfit. If those conditions meant that I could run only 30 seconds before I had to stop to walk, so be it. Third, I would have to make my goals much smaller; I started with 30 seconds. When I felt my body starting to run out of breath, I would walk until I caught my breath again, and then I would slowly run some more. I would then repeat the pattern regardless of how long each run was.

The next day, I would try to make my first run last 31 seconds and so on, until I was able to run the entire mile without stopping to walk. It took me one year to be able to do that. I knew it was longer than it took many people to work up to a mile, but I had accomplished my goal — I had enjoyed myself, I had been active for a year, and I had gotten a bonus — my asthma went away (bet you thought I was going to say I had lost weight). Actually, I did, but that had not been part of the plan. I didn't have to think about losing weight because my body, as the expert, took what I had given it and did the work!

Maybe you feel you need a few more specifics on how to start where you're at to become an active and lean person. Here are a few pointers:

- Come to terms and accept where you're at. Don't set any rules or have any expectations with respect to how you should exercise, when you should exercise, or how soon goals should be met.

- Use self-talk skills. Start thinking in terms of movement, play, or activity, rather than exercise. The brain will find that type of thinking much more appealing and work with you rather than against you.

- Set goals, but make them small ones. The goals need to be small enough to feel doable. If it doesn't feel doable, the goal needs to be smaller.

- Use reinforcement, both in terms of self-talk and actual rewards, for encouragement and incentives to keep playing toward your goals.

- Finally, if you expect the impossible, don't be surprised if you fail. It's helpful and often essential to step back and look at the whole picture before embarking on something. You can inadvertently stack the deck against yourself. Think and study the situation. Find the easiest route to your destination. There's no reason to take the most difficult road.

Chapter 15 Tidbits

- The brain has many negative associations with the word "exercise" and will likely resist your efforts to exercise regularly, as long as you think of it as something that you *have to* do.

- The brain loves to play. In a sense, your brain never grows up. If you convince it that it can play at whatever you want to do, it will follow willingly.

- Goals about exercise are meant to be achieved, but they can't be achieved if they aren't small enough for you to feel that you can accomplish them.

- Goals need to be individualized, because what is a small enough goal for one person may be too big for another.

- Don't complicate things. Take the easiest route to an active and lean lifestyle.

My "Mind Over Fat Matters" Notes

What I want to remember:

What I want to do:

How this will enrich my life:

Chapter 16

The Psychology of Weighing

I'm Not Losing Fast Enough

Should you weigh yourself everyday? Should it be once per week? The number of magazine articles about dieting is endless, and the advice about weighing can be as confusing as the advice about whether we should worry about the number of eggs we eat, whether we should drink a glass of wine each day or totally abstain, or whether we should trust ads about a new drug that "has no significant side effects."

Some experts say that weighing should be kept to a minimum so that we don't get obsessed about it; some say that weighing daily helps prevent us from losing our awareness so that we don't cheat; and others tell us to stay away from weighing all together. Which is the correct advice? How often should we weigh to improve our chances of success with managing our weight throughout our lifetime? Well, would you believe that all of this advice has a grain of truth to it and, at the same time, all of it is wrong?

Most dieters believe that the more you weigh yourself, the more motivated you'll be to lose weight and the faster you will lose it. The typical dieter weighs every day and, sometimes, even several times per day. This dieter usually keeps weight charts and talks a lot about their weight and dieting. He or she has set a specific weight goal.

The brain becomes obsessed with the issue of weight when we make it focus excessively on weight. It's also true that when weight is our primary focus, there is less attention paid to the behaviors that result in our weight. With so much obsessive focus on weight, it becomes too frustrating and anxiety provoking to continue the fight, so the brain starts to feel defeated and gives up. This is when dieters may start avoiding weighing-in or go off their diets. The truth is that less rigidity about weight and weighing-in will spell more success with an individual's weight management.

Americans are, by far, the most weight-conscious culture (literally) that I have come to know. No other people weigh themselves as often or know their exact weight better than Americans, and no other culture is as afraid of weighing-in. Could there be a connection between this and the epidemic of overweight individuals in this country?

If you view weighing-in as a time when you find out if you are a success or a failure, then weighing-in, no matter how frequent, will be a problem. Weighing-in needs to be seen as an opportunity to get some information. However, it's not the most important piece of information that you need concerning your weight management. It's only one of many things that you can use to help yourself achieve your weight goals. If you had the means for reliable information about the actual amount of fat you have lost or how much leaner you've gotten, those would be pieces of information that would be of greater use to you because, after all, it's fat you're trying to work on, not the sum total of what you weigh. Your household scales are not sophisticated enough, however, to give you this kind of information accurately, and to get the information is too costly for most people. Nor could you get this data often enough to be of much help. So you're stuck with your scales and your clothes as *guides* to whether you're going in the right direction with your attempts to lose weight, or if you need to change something. The good news is that it's possible to use a regular, household scale in productive ways that can keep you from making weighing-in a counterproductive exercise.

What is the information that you get when you weigh yourself? The scale tells you what you weigh or the total weight of everything that is inside and on you at the moment that you step on the scale (this assumes also that the scale you're using is accurate). Your total weight would include any clothes you may have on, your hair, organs, muscle, skin, waste, water, blood, etc. — you get the picture. The scale isn't reflecting only fat. If the scale indicates that you've lost weight, you can't know how much of the lost weight is fat, water, muscle, or waste. If the scale indicates that you've gained weight, it still doesn't tell you exactly what it was that you've gained.

Your weight can vary from one day to another or even at different times of the day, even if you're not trying to lose weight. Your weight can vary due to what or how much you've eaten, the time of day when you weigh, how much water you may be retaining (this is especially true of women whose water weight can vary drastically due to their fluctuating hormone levels), or how much muscle mass you may have gained or lost due to exercise or the lack of it. An illness can also cause unusual fluctuations in weight. This doesn't mean the household scale can't be useful to you, but, rather, that you need to view the information it provides realistically and not give the scale more importance than it deserves. You need to deal with weighing-in in a way that won't be counterproductive to your weight-loss plans.

There are several factors that determine the best weighing method for each individual. The first factor is probably the most important. It has to do with attitude or your mental perspective toward the whole issue of weighing-in. Right off the bat, you have to deal with your brain again. If you remember correctly, the brain isn't going to want to do anything that's uncomfortable, so if weighing-in involves being judged or punished in any way, the brain will resist. And that's exactly what weighing-in has come to mean for most people — a time to judge or measure worth. It's important to approach the scale unemotionally. Weighing-in should not be a test; it is simply a tool that you may choose to use to help you achieve something. If you approach the scale with rules in your head such as, "I should have lost weight today. I must lose two pounds this week. I can't gain weight," then you're setting yourself up to fail.

Instead, if you approach the scale calmly and look at it as a tool, you might say something like, "Let's see what the scale shows today. My weight is the same as yesterday. Interesting. Overall, I've been reducing and I'm doing well with my activity level and nutrition, as well as my fat intake. I haven't eaten compulsively for a long time. That's all very good. I'm going in the right direction." Or you might say, "The scale shows my weight as two pounds higher than yesterday. Interesting. I'm still doing well with my behaviors, so it must be something other than fat gain. Let's see. I am close to my period so I may be retaining water. I had a high salt day yesterday that may be contributing, also. I don't know the exact reason, but overall, I'm still doing the right things, so I'll continue with those things. Besides, my reading about how the body loses and gains weight says that I can't have gained two pounds of just fat overnight. My body is more of an expert than I am on how it loses and gains weight. I'll keep doing my job and let it do its job."

This may also be true, "I've been gaining weight consistently the past couple of weeks. I'm still exercising and my nutrition is good. However, I've been eating out more recently and, I have to admit, I've been drinking more and eating more desserts. My body's just reflecting what I'm doing. I guess I'll take a look at this more closely." All three examples show how weigh-ins can be used to your advantage, as tools, rather than as determiners of your success or failure.

The second factor involves having realistic expectations. Remember that your body and brain are better experts than you are about your physiology. They know exactly how fast or slowly you are able to lose fat based on the food and exercise you are providing yourself. However fast or slow the scale or your clothes reflect your weight loss to be, there is a logical reason for it. Rather than getting frustrated or angry at the number reflected on the scale, use that number to help you figure out if your behaviors are on the right track.

Your body will only gain or lose weight at the rate at which it is capable of doing so. You can't change this, so instead of continuing to think that you can decide how fast or slowly you should lose or gain weight, consider yourself as just part of a team with your body and brain. As long as you're doing your part, the other members of the team will do theirs. The speed doesn't matter. It can only happen at the rate that is physiologically possible, considering what you're doing, your heredity, and the laws of nature. That's why it makes no sense to set deadlines for weight loss. It will happen when it *can* happen, so it's best to relax, do the work, and enjoy the ride. The rewards will come; it's a matter of trust in your body and yourself.

The third factor involving weighing-in and successful weight management has to do with having goals that aren't rigid. Your goals, however, should be more about behaviors than a number on the scale. Goals dealing with your activity level, nutrition and food selection, portion control, and priorities deal more directly with things that will cause your fat loss than any number on which you might choose to focus. Besides, unless you're an expert in biochemistry, it's best to stay away from trying to guess what your "right" weight should be. Everyone is different physiologically and it is next to impossible to determine what the best weight is for someone.

If you're going to focus on numbers at all, it makes more sense to think of a weight range, or better yet, think of the lifestyle you wish to have on a long-term basis. For example, let's say that I want a lifestyle where I walk outside everyday for about an hour, take a 10-minute nap every day, have a full-time office job, watch TV for an hour each day, and play tennis once per week. I would then focus on achieving that lifestyle and let my body tell me what weight it can maintain with that lifestyle. If I am not willing to change my lifestyle to one that is going to produce a lower weight, then I have to accept the weight that reflects my lifestyle. On a smaller scale, if I were unwilling to change my daily habit of eating out, then I would have to face that my expectations for a specific weight goal or range might have to be changed.

Finally, regarding how often to weigh yourself, experiment with what works for you. Once your attitude about the scale is based on reality, you can choose to weigh yourself every day, once per week, once per month, or on a varying schedule — if at all. Some people feel they get enough information through their clothes and never weigh themselves. Some people like getting information on a daily basis. It's all up to you. Try out different techniques and choose one you like, knowing that you can change your mind any time you want to do so.

I've had times in my life when I've weighed daily, as well as a two-year period when I didn't weigh at all. The interesting thing is that, regardless of my weighing method, my weight has remained very stable for all the years since I gave up worrying about weight. I've had a great deal of fun, eaten wonderful food, and have been consistently active. I've done my part, my body has rewarded me, and my brain has played along with me. We're a great team!

Chapter 16 Tidbits

- How you view weighing yourself has an impact on your success with managing your weight.

- The weight scale is just a cold, inanimate object that provides a small (and relatively insignificant) amount of information about your total weight. It only tells you how much your entire body weighs at a given moment. It doesn't tell you how much fat you may have lost or gained.

- The more emotional importance that you place on weighing yourself, the more counterproductive weighing will be for you.

- Focus on behaviors, not weight. Keep rules out of it. Be realistic with goals and expectations.

- There are no rules about weighing. You can choose to weigh or not to weigh, and you can change how frequently you weigh — any time you want. Experiment and have fun; just don't lose sight of what really is important — and it's not weighing.

My "Mind Over Fat Matters" Notes

What I want to remember:

What I want to do:

How this will enrich my life:

Chapter 17

Clothes, Shopping, and You

Few people would be surprised that trying on clothes can be a psychological barrier to managing their weight. It's especially difficult in a culture that spells out which clothes sizes are acceptable and which aren't acceptable. It's not easy to be shopping for clothes, find an item you simply love, and go to try it on, only to find that it's too small. "How can that be? It's the same size I always wear. How can I have gained weight? I can't go to a size bigger." Sound familiar?

The attitude that you have when you try on clothes that are too small, don't look good on you, make you look heavier, or are a larger size than you think is considered acceptable, can make or break the best weight-loss plans.

Depending on how you emotionally handle the issues of clothes shopping and trying on clothes, your brain can react with resistance, depression, frustration, and many other emotions that can lead to overeating or eating compulsively. If you dread shopping for clothes or trying them on, it's a clue that your thinking about weight has become a psychological barrier to your success with managing weight.

Let's stop for a minute and think about what clothes may mean to other people around the world. Some cultures wear a lot of clothes, like Eskimos, others wear very little clothing, like people from hot climates who may wear as little as a small piece of material covering only the genitals. The majority of people wear clothes for protection or to decorate their bodies. In both these cases, clothing provides something positive.

In most cultures you would be hard-pressed to find someone who uses clothing to define her worth as a person. It is when you cross that line and allow what you wear or what size you wear to determine how good you are, or how you should be feeling, that you run into problems. Just like with that cold, inanimate object — the bathroom scale — clothes ought not to have power over you. Clothing should instead serve to make you physically comfortable and add little bonuses to your life through the variety of colors available and their ability to enhance your appearance.

You can always choose to look better than you do or worse than you do. Clothes are tools for looking better if that's what you wish — but that's all they are, tools. They do not make you acceptable or unacceptable.

Some people are more interested in the way clothes appeal to their senses. These are the folks that we might think dress weird or eccentrically. They simply get into the textures, colors, and other qualities of the clothing, rather than how the clothing actually makes them look.

Other people are really into putting clothing together so that it enhances their best features and de-emphasizes others. These are usually the people we think of as quite stylish. There is nothing wrong with either approach.

The problem comes in when you have rules about clothing that says such things as, "I must never wear anything bigger than a size _____." "I must always be a size _____." "I must never let anyone know that I wear a size _____." Having these kinds of rules alone makes you uptight. Being afraid or ashamed of your size is no way to live life happily and comfortably. As a matter of fact, the more rules you have about your clothes size and trying on clothes, the more tension you produce in yourself. What have you learned about stress and tension? It can lead to overeating, compulsive eating, and wanting to give up on your goals.

Instead, the whole issue of clothing needs to be looked at in a neutral fashion. You need to have a supportive, encouraging, and loving approach with yourself when it comes to your clothes. Treat yourself as if you were your own best friend. You wouldn't say to your loved friend, "Oh, my gosh, you can't be a bigger size. You shouldn't be more than a size eight. What's wrong with you? You should be ashamed of yourself." You wouldn't judge your dear friend by her pant size, or how she looked in a particular outfit. You would just love her, want her to be happy, and be encouraging of her efforts at looking her best while enjoying life. So it should be with all of us.

It's time to throw away rules about clothes sizes and those of society in general. Have fun shopping. The goal with shopping for and trying on clothes needs to be to find the items that fit comfortably and look the most flattering, regardless of their size.

Did you know that when your clothes are too tight, you tend to be more aware of your body? If you're uncomfortable and more aware of your body, doesn't it make sense that you might obsess more about your body? Tight clothes make you feel bigger, no matter what size you are. So it makes more sense that if you want to obsess less about your body and feel more relaxed so that you can focus on other things, while still making headway with your weight goals, you should wear clothes that are comfortably looser (forgetting the size number).

Here's another interesting fact. There is no standard for clothes sizes. That's why sometimes you can fit well into your usual size while other times (even on the same day or the same store) you have to take a size bigger or smaller. Each manufacturer has their standards for sizes. Even then, you may find differences between different items of the same size from the same manufacturer. So, if you're going to have rules about sizes, shopping, and fitting, get ready to drive yourself crazy.

Recently I watched a television special that discussed how today's clothing sizes are bigger than they were 20 years ago. That's right. Today's size 4 is not the same size 4 of 20 years past. It's bigger. It's a marketing ploy. Clothing manufacturers know that Americans are heavier today than they used to be and that they're not likely to buy an article of clothing that is a bigger size than they used to wear. The solution? Just put a number "8" on what used to be a "10" or a "12." That will make the consumer happy and a happy consumer is one who consumes.

If you don't have rules about clothes shopping, that means that you don't have to buy something just because you're shopping. You don't have to always find something that fits or that you like. With no rules, shopping and trying on clothes becomes playtime. Remember playing dress up? You didn't worry about anything then except having fun. Wow, just think. Here's another opportunity to have more playtime in your adult life. All right!

So, if trying on clothes isn't fun and you can see that you put too much meaning into your clothing size, you can consider your thinking about these things as a psychological barrier to managing your weight successfully. Here's how to change that:

- Start paying attention to what you say to yourself when you are dressing, shopping for clothes, or thinking about your clothes size. Pick out the rules and other illogical thoughts.

- Point out to yourself why your thoughts are illogical or self-defeating.

- After disputing your illogical thoughts, purposely replace the old thoughts with thoughts that are positive, logical, and are going to help you manage weight more successfully.

- Point out to yourself why these new thoughts are going to make your life better and more fun.

- Reinforce yourself for catching the self-defeating thinking, and make a commitment to consistently dispute such thoughts in the future so that you can eliminate them permanently.

- Imagine yourself as a child playing dress-up and having fun.

You really only need clothes for shelter, but you also can have the luxury of having clothes as play tools. They aren't living, breathing beings that are out to get you!

Chapter 17 Tidbits

- The way you think about trying on and shopping for clothes can become a psychological barrier to your success with weight.

- When you have rules about your clothes size and judge yourself according to these rules, you cause tension and other emotions that will get in the way of your best intentions. Breaking a diet and compulsively eating because you're upset after trying on clothes is not an uncommon occurrence.

- Clothes are meant for comfort and to add a little spice to your life — nothing more. Have fun with the process of selecting clothes. This will manage your weight successfully and make your life more pleasant in general.

- Treat clothes like you did as a child. Play with them. Play dress-up, get into colors, textures, and styles for the fun of it, and don't let anyone make you wear anything that's not comfortable.

- Tight clothes can make you obsess about your body more. They can make you feel bigger than you are. Wearing clothes that are comfortable keeps your focus on other, more productive things that lead to better weight management.

My "Mind Over Fat Matters" Notes

What I want to remember:

What I want to do:

How this will enrich my life:

Chapter 18

Your Body and You:

Improving Body Image

Body image is the perception of one's body with respect to size, attractiveness, and worth. Depending on that perception and your belief system, you develop emotional responses to your body. These responses can be negative or positive, depending on your body image and judgment of that image. For example, if I perceive my size as large and my attractiveness as plain, and I believe that large, plain bodies are bad, unacceptable, or worthless, I would have negative feelings about my body. In perceiving my body, I might find myself saying things like, "I'm so fat. I can't stand myself. I'm fat and ugly. No one will be attracted to me because of my body."

On the other hand, if I perceive myself as large and plain but believe that large and plain are acceptable, I might find myself saying, "This outfit looks good on me. I look best in solid colors, and red is an especially good color for my rather average features. I'll go with that." In these examples, both people view their bodies fairly equally, but judge them differently.

When a person perceives her body as being significantly different than it looks in reality, we say that the person has a "distorted body image." The truth is that everyone distorts to some extent when perceiving his or her body. We can't help it because it is impossible for us to view ourselves from the perspective that others have of us. We view ourselves from within ourselves. Others view us from without. The closest we can get to viewing ourselves the way that others do is by looking in a mirror. Yet, there is still some distortion when we look at ourselves in a mirror. Other people will always have a more objective view of our appearance than we do. That is why other people can be better judges of how we look than we are.

It's also true that some of us distort our body image more than others. When we have a positive body image, it means that we generally feel good or are, at least, accepting and loving about our body. When we have a negative body image, we are usually critical and rejecting of our body. Most chronic dieters, regardless of their actual size, have a negative body image, and some of these mistakenly believe that being critical of their body is somehow going to motivate them to do better. Wrong! The fact is that, regardless of one's body size or shape, the more positive the body image, the more successful one will be with losing and managing weight.

Why does a negative body image spell failure so often? Strangely enough, the brain influences one to behave in ways that are consistent with one's body image. If you have a negative body image, it would be inconsistent to do things that make you feel comfortable, relaxed, and encouraged. The negative body image is only consistent with behaviors that instead make you feel anxious, discouraged, and frustrated. As you've already learned, negative emotions make it next to impossible to keep up all the behaviors that will lead to your success with your weight. A negative body image will do the same. It leads to failure in achieving permanent weight loss. It requires a positive body image to be able to consistently follow behaviors, such as exercising regularly and eating healthily, that will produce permanent weight loss. So it behooves you to do all that you can to come to terms with your body — accept it, treat it well, pamper it, do nice things for it, decorate it, and have fun with it. All these lead to a positive body image.

Accepting your body does not mean that you will be unmotivated to make changes, or that you don't care what it looks like. If you love someone, a friend, perhaps, you want her to be happy and you like her to want to look her best. You are pleased when she looks the best she can look. However, you accept her limitations physically and don't expect more than what is possible for her. You also don't judge her worth by what she looks like. It is the same with your own body. You want to have the desire to look the best that you can, not because it is expected of you, but because you love yourself and know that taking care of your body and helping it to look its best adds to the quality of your life and your happiness. When you look your best, it has a domino effect — you want other things to be better, also. It's motivating.

If there's something that is impossible to change, like the shape of your face or your general body proportions, you don't waste time expecting these things to be completely different. Don't waste time on the impossible. Do spend time on the possible. If it's possible to change the appearance of a characteristic of the face through a different hairstyle, by all means try it. If certain styles or colors of clothes look better than others, then use them. It's also true that if you especially like something, if it brings you pleasure, but it's not something that makes you look your best, then who cares? It's more important to please yourself in this type of situation than it is to please others.

I'll never forget a very talented woman I once met in my office. Susan had a thing for clothes from the 1950s. That's practically all she wore. She was definitely out of style and some of the clothes weren't particularly flattering, but it was apparent that wearing them made her everyday life more fun. Who's to argue with that? Her body image was so positive that it didn't matter at all what she looked like to others, she was pleased and that was what mattered. So, the bottom line is, look your best and feel your best, but make feeling your best the bigger priority.

Here are two good examples of looking your best. When I was a graduate student and doing research on eating disorders, I attended an Overeaters Anonymous meeting. I sat down at a large, round table, around which were many very large, round women. One woman in particular caught my eye. She happened to be the one leading the group that night. She was, without a doubt, one of the largest women there, but what was most noticeable about her was not her size. She had done the most wonderful job of looking her best that I had ever seen (so much so that I've never forgotten her). You could tell that she had carefully selected her clothing to enhance her best features without just trying to hide her size. The colors, textures, accessories, and lines of her clothes gave her an overall pleasing appearance. She was attractive because of the type of loving attention she had paid to herself. Aside from that, she had great posture, holding herself with pride. She showed confidence through good eye contact with others and spoke with assurance. For years I've used her example to demonstrate the choices we have no matter what size or shape we are.

Jackie, on the other hand, was another story. Jackie came to my office for the first time looking like a balloon. She was slightly overweight but definitely not obese. Jackie, however, felt she was the biggest woman alive. Because of this body image, she struggled to hide her body entirely. Unfortunately, she tried to do this by wearing huge sweatpants and the biggest sweatshirt I had ever seen. She looked like the Pillsbury Doughboy. This is what she wore every session for several weeks. One of the first things we worked on, as you might guess, was her body image. After several trying weeks, Jackie finally came to a session dressed with more pride. It was an amazing transformation. Jackie was actually thinner than I had thought. The billowy sweat clothes had made her look bigger instead of hiding her fat. Jackie never wore her sweatsuit again and she learned that people on the outside (in this case, me) were going to be more objective about her size than she was (at least until she learned to accept herself completely).

A negative body image will be a definite psychological barrier to managing weight for a lifetime. The brain, burdened with a poor body image, will compel a person to behave in ways that result in weight gain rather than loss. After all, if you believe that you're fat, ugly, and unsuccessful, you can't possibly do things that are positive, that wouldn't fit with the body image. No, a poor body image goes with things like negative emotions, compulsive eating, inactivity, and poor eating habits. If you want to do the things that lead to fitness, you have to have a good image of yourself, feel good about who you are and your efforts. That will lead to behaviors that are consistent with your image of yourself. Then you'll find yourself wanting to be active, caring about what you eat, and being excited about everything you do along the way to leanness.

So, how do you know if your body image is a problem, and how would you eliminate this type of problem? The first question is an easy one to answer; the second is a bit more complicated, yet not as difficult as one would expect.

Body image is a problem if you…

- …worry a lot about what others think of your body.

- …feel ashamed about any part of your body.

- …judge your acceptability as a person on how your body looks.

- …spend an inordinate amount of time judging other people's bodies.

- …don't feel warm feelings of acceptance when you think of your body.

- …believe there are only certain body shapes that are acceptable, and that yours certainly isn't one of them.

- …get feelings of anger, frustration, or anxiety when thinking about your body or looking at your body in a mirror.

- …avoid looking at yourself in a mirror.

- …believe that you cannot be acceptable until you reach certain weight goals.

- …feel obsessed with your body.

How do you eliminate a poor body image and learn to accept your body? First, it's important to realize that you have been mistaken. Your negative body image has not made you more motivated and it is not going to help you achieve changes in your weight and body size. It will not make the impossible, possible, by changing inherited traits like the basic proportions of your body. Just as you cannot become taller or shorter, or have bigger or smaller feet just because you want them, you cannot change your basic body type.

Second, you need to start treating yourself as you would treat a loved one. You love your loved ones as they are. You do not require that they all be attractive, thin, and rich in order for you to give them your love. As a matter of fact, when you love someone, you usually concentrate on and notice special things about them that you feel supersede their general appearance. It might be the way they laugh, their kindness, their curly hair, or their cute walk. You love them as they are and appreciate them for their unique qualities. That's the way you need to practice treating yourself; however, it does take practice. Your expectations for change have to be realistic. At first, you may catch yourself many times treating yourself in the old unloving way, but that's the time to stop and consciously act in an accepting and loving manner.

Third, pay close attention to comparisons. Comparing yourself with others is just asking for problems. That leads nowhere, except maybe straight to the refrigerator. Comparing is a useless exercise. It accomplishes nothing unless you actually want to punish yourself and make yourself feel as badly as possible. Then comparing is definitely the road you want to take. Catch yourself whenever you're comparing yourself to someone else and say, "Oops, that's never brought me anything good. I don't need to do that any more. It's never gotten me anywhere. Everyone is unique and acceptable. I may have goals about my weight, but weight is not the center of my life and doesn't determine my worth as a person. Having a good body image is what is going to help me accomplish my goals, and comparing myself to others isn't going to help me have a positive body image." Afterwards, point out all the good and nice things about yourself and your efforts. Say something loving and move on.

Fourth, don't call yourself derogatory names (like stupid, dumb, jerk, or idiot). Don't fool yourself into thinking that you're just kidding or playing. Remember, your brain is listening. This is a practice everyone can do without regardless of the reason.

Fifth, do special things for yourself on a regular basis. Think about the thoughtful things you often think to do for people you like. Do them for yourself. If doing thoughtful things for others makes them feel good, doing them for yourself will make you feel good, too.

Sixth, use positive self-talk (does this sound like a déjà vu?). When referring to yourself, focus on always using the positive. For example, instead of saying, "I haven't reached my goal yet," say, "I'm still progressing toward my goal." Instead of, "This shirt makes me look fat," point out, "I think the other shirt is more flattering on me." In neither case are you lying to yourself; you're only focusing on the positive rather than the negative and staying away from your psychological barriers.

Finally, it's important to practice looking at your body as a whole rather than looking at it as parts. Have you ever noticed how television commercials treat the female body as parts? Do an experiment. Compare commercials featuring females as opposed to those featuring males. Notice how often the female body is presented first as a part (the camera will start with a close-up of breasts, groin, eye, hair, or legs before zooming out to the whole figure, if it zooms at all). How often do they do the same with the male body? We'll never know which came first. Many women tend to treat their bodies in the same way — as parts. These women think of themselves as the parts that they dislike the most, focusing on their butts, hips, arms, or thighs, instead of the *gestalt,* or the whole. Just the opposite is true when other people look at us. They perceive us as a whole unit rather than as parts. We do the same with them. Think about it.

An interesting sociological study was done a number of years ago comparing men and women. It was found that when men think about their bodies, they tend to focus on aspects of their body that they like, or ascribe positive characteristics to unusual features such as their big feet, their pot belly, or their big ears. Women tended to do the opposite. They focused on the features that they liked the least, and tended to criticize or downplay even their more attractive features. They found that women tended to undervalue their good points and overvalue their lesser points. Interesting, isn't it?

Remember what it was like as a very young child? We were barely aware of our bodies. We had more important things on our minds, such as going about the business of enjoying life. There was never any reason to change that. Let's go back to focusing more on using our bodies to help us enjoy life and less on putting our bodies down when they're only trying to help us.

I once bluntly asked a patient who had exhausted me with her attempts to convince me that her body must be rejected, the following question: "Okay, I understand that you feel you have hugely fat legs. Would you rather have those hugely fat legs or no legs at all?" She finally stopped and thought. "I'd rather have the legs, but…" I quickly said, "Wait, you have choices in life to be happier or less happy in any given situation. You have inherited legs that are proportionately bigger than you would like. You can change some things about them but there are limits to what you can do. You either accept the legs, do whatever you can to improve their condition, or make yourself miserable for the rest of your life. If you choose the latter, you will have sacrificed your entire life for something that, in the greater scheme of things, is small stuff. What do your hugely fat legs do that help you enjoy life better than if you didn't have the legs at all?" Reluctantly, she said, "They help me walk, sit, stand, get into bed, get to wherever I want…yeah, yeah, I get it." She put up a good fight, but eventually she did get it and moved on with life with the help of her less than hugely fat legs (that's because she started focusing on shaping them up rather than complaining about them).

Your body image is an important ingredient in the recipe for a comfortable existence with your body and for making weight management an uncomplicated process. It's worth the time it takes to find out if your body image is a psychological barrier to your success with fitness and to end the barrier, if it exists.

Chapter 18 Tidbits

- The brain influences you to behave in ways that are consistent with your body image. If you have a negative body image, you will not be doing things that make you feel encouraged, motivated, and relaxed. It requires a positive body image to make you want to do things that are going to lead to weight loss, like physical activity and eating well.

- Many dieters have a negative body image and believe that using criticism and judging themselves will somehow motivate them to do better. Just the opposite is true.

- In achieving a positive body image, there are dos and don'ts. Don't compare yourself to others and don't call yourself derogatory names. Do special things for yourself on a regular basis, use positive self-talk, and look at your body as a whole, not as parts.

- Accepting your body does not mean that you will be unmotivated to make changes, or that you don't care what it looks like. Love yourself and know that taking care of your body and helping it to look its best adds to the quality of your life and your happiness.

- Take a childlike attitude about your body. Use it to help you enjoy life and, beyond that, give it little thought.

My "Mind Over Fat Matters" Notes

What I want to remember:

What I want to do:

How this will enrich my life:

Chapter 19

"I Am Ashamed of Myself":

Dealing With Guilt and

Learning Compassion

Feeling guilt and shame about oneself is one of the biggest obstacles to losing weight successfully. Yet, guilt is one of the most common problems that dieters have to deal with. Our culture believes that guilt and shame are motivating factors, and since motivation is deemed to be essential in dieting, it must mean that guilt must also be a part of a plan to lose weight. In fact, it is one of the most destructive and unproductive things you can do to yourself. This psychological barrier alone can make the best weight-loss plan fail royally.

Basically, at the bottom of guilt and shame are rules that say that if you don't do what you set out to do (perfectly), you should feel guilty because you have done something terribly wrong and worthy of feeling shame. By feeling this guilt and shame, you are supposed to want to do better or make sure not to repeat the wrongdoing. If this really happened, our world would be a much better place because the majority of us are quite adept at feeling guilt. Few people are incapable of feeling guilt. Such people are called sociopaths.

Sociopaths are what are commonly known as "cons." They feel no guilt to trip them up, so they're usually quite good at "pulling the wool over people's eyes." Most of them are in prisons.

It's impossible, however, to ever become a person that feels no guilt at all. Guilt is a normal human emotion, albeit, not a very useful one. There are, however, two other emotions that are related to guilt that do serve useful purposes and help us through life's journey. These two emotions are concern and remorse. When we feel concern and remorse, we recognize that we have done something wrong or that our behavior has caused a problem, and we want to correct the problem or make-up for the wrongdoing. The difference between concern and remorse versus guilt and shame is that only with guilt and shame do we cross the line toward judging our personal worth. Guilt and shame affect our self-esteem. When we feel these emotions, we view ourselves as having less personal worth, we think of ourselves as "bad" because we did what we did. With concern and remorse, we only view the BEHAVIOR as wrong or bad. We never cross over to our self-esteem.

The reason why guilt and shame aren't motivating emotions is because we tend to get stuck once we put our self-esteem down. We become obsessed with how bad or unworthy we are, so we can't break away from that long enough or quickly enough to start actually doing something about the situation that went wrong. People who suffer from guilt and shame tend to "stew in their own juice." It's paralyzing. And the longer we stew in our juice from guilt, the worse we feel about ourselves because while we're stewing, we're not correcting anything, so we have even more to feel guilty about.

Concern and remorse are motivating because, since they don't touch our self-esteem, we still feel good about ourselves. We still believe in our abilities and ourselves. We still feel worthy of good things in life. We're not depressed or "down-in-the-dumps." That means we still have the energy and we still want to see things better again. That's motivation.

There should never be a concern about not feeling guilty because the less guilt you feel, the more you'll accomplish in life. With respect to your purpose here — managing your weight for a lifetime — the less guilt and shame you feel about your weight or efforts to lose it, the more successful you'll be with it all. Remember, concern/remorse — yes; guilt/shame — no!

Guilt and shame create negative emotions such as frustration, anger, and anxiety. The brain has never responded well to such emotions. These extreme negative emotions only serve to paralyze you and preoccupy the brain with things that aren't going to get you out of the predicament you're in. In addition, guilt and shame go hand-in-hand with low self-esteem. You've learned that the brain leads you to act in keeping with your self-esteem. Therefore, when you feel guilt and shame, the brain will compel you to behave in ways

that are consistent with low self-esteem. That means you will have little motivation to do positive things and keep trying to improve. You won't want
to exercise, eat well, problem-solve, and all the other things necessary to accomplish your goal of managing your weight successfully for the rest of your
life. Guilt and shame aren't responsible reactions to setbacks, contrary to the
thinking of many dieters. They will not motivate you to do better and will
not prevent you from falling again.

A more responsible and effective reaction to setbacks is compassion.
You've learned previously how compassion can make others feel better and
encouraged to go forward with challenges. We've discussed how people's
learning can be affected negatively when they are confronted with criticism
and judgment, and enhanced when given compassion. This phenomenon
works the same with you. If you fall and beat yourself up about it, you'll fall
more often. If, instead, when you fall, you treat yourself with compassion,
you'll feel light enough to pick yourself back up and continue to try.

What do compassion and criticism sound like when you talk with yourself? Like this: Criticism: *I can't believe I just did that. How many times do I
have to keep messing up? I'm just a failure and big stupid jerk. I'll never get any
better at this.* Compassion: *Oops! I've made that mistake before. What happened
this time that I didn't see it coming? I need to look at this more closely to see what
I can do to make it less likely to happen again. It's okay, though. My intentions
are good, I'm trying, and I've accomplished quite a bit already. Look at all that
I've been changing. Besides, change only happens one step at a time. I'm not going
to get down about this, but, instead, I'm going to study it and see what I can do
about it.*

Guilt and shame will always be psychological barriers. You know you're
suffering from them if:

- You tend to call yourself derogatory names whenever you feel you've
  messed up.

- You seem to lose motivation whenever you make mistakes.

- You find yourself unable to come out of obsessing over your mistake
  and feel paralyzed by it.

- You easily give up when you've accidentally failed at something.

The solution to eliminating guilt and shame is learning to be compassionate with yourself. If you ever have any trouble coming up with what the
compassionate response should be to something, think of how you would
respond to someone you love and respect when they have made a mistake.

Then do the same with yourself. Study the problem as if it were a project you were given to solve at work. Find the kinks and develop a plan for getting rid of them. Set up new goals to work on the kinks without rules. Don't forget to have rewards for effort and for reaching goals. Focus more on what has been accomplished rather than what has not. Finally, allow yourself to celebrate like a child when you've worked out the kinks.

Chapter 19 Tidbits

- Guilt and shame are two of the biggest obstacles to losing weight successfully.

- Guilt and shame lead to emotions that only make you stew in your juice, feel unmotivated, and make you want to quit.

- Contrary to what many dieters think, guilt and shame are not responsible reactions to setbacks and do not prevent you from falling again.

- Compassion, not guilt and shame, provides you with a way to handle setbacks. It increases motivation, prevents loss of self-esteem, and helps correct the problem that caused the setback in the first place.

My "Mind Over Fat Matters" Notes

What I want to remember:

What I want to do:

How this will enrich my life:

Chapter 20

"Who Am I?":

Learning About Yourself

You've probably heard the saying that knowledge is power. It's true, and knowledge about oneself is definite power — brain power. The more you know and understand about how you tick, the better your brain will be at helping you through all the challenges in your life. It's especially true when it comes to anything having to do with making changes in your eating and fitness world. It can make your psychological barriers come to light and it highlights the direction you need to take when you encounter a stumbling block. In addition, it gives confidence because you become the expert, the expert about what works with you.

As a therapist, I tell my clients that my job is to help them become their own therapist so that they won't need me any more. This is accomplished by helping them to understand themselves, their strengths and weaknesses, and what works and doesn't work for them as individuals. I know when my job is coming to an end when the client starts consistently coming to sessions reporting the challenges they encountered and how they solved them as opposed to bringing a problem for me to solve.

In the world of dieting, people have been taught to look for answers from outside themselves. They focus on the concrete side of things, like trying to follow recipes, diets, and exercise plans in books, magazines, and designed by diet gurus. Although there certainly are some basic fundamentals of activity, nutrition, and weight loss that can be learned from outside sources, the major keys to being fit for a lifetime come from knowing ourselves enough to know how to apply those basics in a way that will work.

Trying to lose weight is as much a psychological issue as it is a physiological one. If your brain is focusing only on the physiological, that leaves all the psychological barriers to get in the way of your efforts. When new clients come into my office asking for a diet or exercise program, I tell them, "I will not be giving you diets or exercise programs. Those you know how to get because you've done it many times before. I will be teaching you how to apply a lot of what you've learned so that it finally works. I will also be teaching you what doesn't work. After I help you to understand what works for you as a unique individual, you'll know exactly what to do."

You're being introspective when you try to look within you to discover what it is about yourself that is causing your behavior. Instead of going through life on automatic pilot, you try to define the feelings you're having and question why you're having those feelings. You explore your history for clues. Perhaps a loved one lied to you when you were a child and now you have trouble feeling trust when people make promises. Maybe you're afraid of taking risks because you were given the message as a child that you weren't capable of figuring things out on your own.

Practicing introspection is one of the best ways to get to know yourself. It's similar to what you do when you've just met someone new and you want to get to know him or her better. You start with asking them questions about themselves, their likes, dislikes, their childhood, and their experiences. If you want to continue to get to know them, you spend time with them and you listen. That would be the equivalent of allowing some alone time or solitude into your life. It's difficult to listen carefully to yourself if you're always around other people. Some people are like that; they're afraid of being alone and go to great lengths to avoid it. Instead, they should make time to be alone and confront whatever fears are making them avoid it. Without this time, some of your most important conflicts in life are never resolved.

It never ceases to amaze me how so many people go through life in continual fear that there will be a moment when they will find themselves alone and thinking. These people are missing some valuable things about life. Not only will they never experience feeling totally at peace with themselves (the only person that will be with them 24 hours per day for the rest of their lives), but they will miss lots of flowers they could have smelled (lying in a hammock in the breeze with birds chirping in the background, smelling the aroma of freshly-opened wisteria flowers with your eyes closed and remembering a special time as a child, sitting and petting your cat while appreciating the silence surrounding you). How do you really get to know someone if you don't spend quality time with them?

So, here are some ways to be more introspective:

- Just for practice, several times a day, ask yourself how you feel at that moment. Don't just answer, "I feel good" or "I feel bad" or "I feel okay." Label the feeling. Do you feel content, sad, bored, anxious, frustrated, jovial, depressed, angry, worthless, or happy? If you can't come up with the exact emotion, find the emotion that comes closet to the one you feel. With practice, it will become easier and faster to come up with the emotions you're feeling at any given time.

- If you're feeling badly, that's the most important time to pay attention and figure out what the emotion is. Do you feel badly because you're feeling hurt, irritated, afraid, enraged, sad, abandoned, or anxious?

- Once you have figured out the emotion that comes closest to what you're feeling, ask yourself, "What is it that made me feel this way right now?" Try to find the trigger for the emotion. Was it something someone said, a mistake you made, a thought, an event, or something someone did?

- Once you have the trigger for the emotion, it's time to figure out when in the past you have had similar feelings. Then try to find the common denominator between those times in your life that you've felt the same way. For example, let's say that your friend canceled a get-together and you found yourself feeling hurt. You may recall that in the past you've felt this way many times, and usually it has to do with people disappointing you by changing their minds about some commitment they made with you. You find that despite their reasons for breaking the commitment, you take it personally.

- Now try to find the situation in childhood where you first felt this way. Perhaps your mother had told you that she would take you to a special place when you were 10 years old. Maybe you had looked forward to this time when you and your mother would spend time alone together, especially since your brother had recently been born and he had been getting most of the attention lately. The special day came but your baby brother was sick so your mother told you the date would have to be postponed, but the date never happened.

Bingo! Now as an adult, when situations happen that remind you (unconsciously) of the forgotten special date with your mother, you get the same feelings of deep hurt.

There are certain types of feelings that will crop up in your life over and over again. It is these feelings that you should be the most concerned about because they're connected like a string of beads to each other, and lead back to a single event that had a lifetime impact on you. Before you can do much about these feelings, you need to be able to define the feelings and know where they originated. You don't have to worry about perfection here. You don't always get a clear picture of what started the ball rolling but, the more you use introspection, the clearer things get. Eventually, things that were so puzzling at one time now make tons of sense. You might find yourself saying something like, "There's that familiar feeling again. Jeff had a perfectly rational reason for canceling and it had nothing to do with not wanting to be with me. This feeling comes from way back and has nothing to do with Jeff and me."

Knowing and understanding your behavior and thinking makes it possible for you to figure out your biggest psychological barriers, and to be more creative in finding solutions to combat these barriers. For example, once you know that one of your biggest psychological issues in life is fear of failure, you can: 1) brainstorm about how to confront this fear; 2) recognize when the fear of failure is interfering with your intentions; 3) decipher the thoughts that are fueling the fear of failure; 4) dispute those irrational thoughts; 5) replace those thoughts with more realistic and logical ones; and 6) come up with incentives to help push you to take the necessary risk so that you will see there was nothing to fear.

Just like a scientist, however, once you've studied something (in this case, yourself), it's time to experiment. Using the knowledge newly attained about your emotional and psychological tendencies, you logically come up with possible solutions. It would be unrealistic to think, however, that the first thing you tried and the first time you tried it, you'd be successful. Experimenting is an opportunity to fine tune things along the way. A good scientist would pick out what worked and what did not work in the first experiment; he or she would then hypothesize why something did or didn't work, and come up with the next experiment based on this information. The second experiment would reveal more important information and opportunities to discard what didn't work and keep what did. Eventually, the working solution would be discovered.

Acceptance is a big part of getting to know and understand yourself. Without acceptance, you would be afraid to look within long enough to find out who you are. You have to be ready to accept the person you're going to explore before you move ahead. If you don't, you'll be blocked time and time again by the judgments and criticisms of all that you'll find. Taking the attitude of discovery is a good counter to any tendency to be judgmental of yourself. In trying to get to know yourself, you're simply looking to see what mysteries and interesting and unique things you'll find. No one else is like you, no one ticks like you do, and no one can become a better expert on you than yourself if you go about it with love, compassion, interest, and the excitement of discovery.

Chapter 20 Tidbits

- Knowledge about yourself is power — power to discover what works and doesn't work for you.

- Introspection is the first step to getting to know how you tick.

- Knowing yourself makes it possible to be more creative in choosing things that work for you. Experimenting with these methods allows you to fine-tune them, discarding what doesn't work well and keeping what does.

- Accept your uniqueness in order to get to know yourself. If you don't accept who you are, you create a psychological barrier to learning how you tick and finding the solutions to your other psychological barriers.

My "Mind Over Fat Matters" Notes

What I want to remember:

What I want to do:

How this will enrich my life:

Chapter 21

"Do I Have an Eating Disorder?"

An eating disorder is a serious matter. In spite of the fact that eating disorders are relatively common these days, unfortunately, that doesn't negate the fact that an eating disorder isn't something to be taken lightly. Having an eating disorder at worst can cost a life, and at least can affect your health and destroy your life emotionally and socially.

So what is an eating disorder? Most people think of someone with an eating disorder as someone who either tries to starve herself or binges on food and throws up. The eating-disordered person is viewed as someone who just wants to be thin. There's a lot more to it than that. The person with an eating disorder is obsessed with weight to the point of making it the most important thing in her life. Because she feels it is the most important thing in her life, she's willing to do just about anything to achieve perfection with her weight. Unfortunately, this person also distorts what she looks like to a severe degree. No matter how far she goes with losing weight or achieving her weight goals, she continues to see huge imperfections and finds herself still falling short of where she feels she needs to be in her efforts. She continues trying harder and harder, becoming more extreme with the methods to achieve perfection.

At the bottom of all this is a person with low self-esteem. This person believes that she has little or no worth as a person unless she achieves perfection, particularly with appearance and weight. This is the type of person who tries to be perfect in other ways, also. She's usually described as an individual who is the perfect student, the perfect friend, or the perfect employee. She often keeps negative emotions in because she doesn't wish to show imperfections in her personality and fears not being liked by others.

Anger is an emotion that someone with an eating disorder tends to have particular difficulty acknowledging. He isn't comfortable with his own anger or that of others, so he has difficulty admitting that he is angry, even to himself.

The most common eating disorders are anorexia, bulimia, and compulsive overeating. The three disorders have more in common than they have differences. The anorexic is thought of as someone who has starved herself to an alarmingly low weight. The anorexic, however, was anorexic way before she got down to her abnormally low weight. The anorexia was what caused her to get into such a state. This is one of the unfortunate things about eating disorders. With our society being so focused on physical appearance and thinness, many victims of eating disorders aren't detected until the condition is severe. Up until then, many are seen as normal people just wanting to look their best. In some cases, they're even admired and reinforced for their self-destructive behaviors of strict dieting and constant attention to their appearance.

Many times I've seen parents in tears, recounting stories of how they had praised their child for dieting, losing weight, or exercising, only to find out when the child couldn't control the dieting, losing weight, or exercising; when the child's health was compromised; when their child lost their social life; that they had lost total control as parents and that their child was in grave danger.

The anorexic fixates on losing weight and controls her eating to whatever extent she deems necessary to achieve her weight goal. Her weight goals are unrealistic to begin with, but even if she achieves her goal, the anorexic will feel she needs to lose more weight and continues to do so. With respect to food, the focus of the anorexic is to eat as little of it as possible. Oftentimes, the anorexic develops rituals with food and sometimes other things, such as exercise. She may count the number of peas on her plate, she may eat the food on her plate counterclockwise, or she may only eat off of certain plates, believing that her rituals help her to maintain control over her eating. At the point when she starts getting pressure from other people to stop losing weight or to eat more, the anorexic becomes more and more secretive and she can be rather good at this. Parents, spouses, and even therapists are often amazed at the things they didn't know the anorexic was doing to keep anyone from interfering with her pursuit of thinness.

With bulimia, although the same pursuit of thinness is being sought, the person, for whatever reason, isn't able to maintain the control over food for long. The bulimic lives through cycles of dieting, binging on food, and then using some form of purging in an attempt to get rid of the huge amounts eaten during the binge. A binge is when someone is trying not to eat, then feels that she's lost control over her eating. She goes straight for the foods that she has been trying to control. The eating itself is rapid and void of savoring. The binger feels frantic while eating and doesn't enjoy the process in the least. Some people even report that while binging, they feel themselves in a sort of trance state. The eating continues compulsively, until either no more food can physically be fit inside the stomach, or someone interrupts them. At such a time, the binger stops, not because she wants to, but because she feels shame about what she does and doesn't want anyone to see her doing it. During the binge, the person does not feel relaxed at all. Remember, this isn't a pleasant event. The binge is accompanied by feelings of fear, anger, frustration, anxiety, depression, or any combination of these. The binge is followed with more negative feelings of shame, guilt, frustration, fear, anger, and self-loathing.

After something like this, it stands to reason that the person would want to get rid of any traces of what she just did. That's where the purge comes in. Many people think that purging means vomiting. Although vomiting can be a form of purging, it isn't the only purge that a person with an eating disorder can use. Some other forms of purging include the use of dieting, laxatives, exercise, and diuretics. A purge is something that is used immediately after a binge for the purpose of compensating for or negating the effects of the binge. With a purge, the person is trying to get rid of the food she binged on. The most direct approach, most obviously, would be to make oneself vomit after the binge.

With excessive exercise, the binger is thinking that she is getting rid of the food by burning up the calories that were contained in the binged food. By strict dieting or fasting, the person is trying to reach a calorie balance through causing a deficit in calories for a while.

Laxatives and diuretics are an even more indirect and irrational method. The individual with an eating disorder believes that weight equals fat. So, whatever she weighs that day equals how fat her body is; therefore, causing the scale or weight to go down means she has lost fat, the fat that was caused by the binge. Another way that the binger who uses laxatives or diuretics thinks is that if she feels thinner, she is less fat. Laxative and diuretic use causes loss of fluids and waste from the body. This causes a deceiving and temporary loss of weight, but, it's water weight, not fat. All of the purging methods are wrought with dangers, including malnutrition, osteoporosis, dental decay, heart problems, and, in some cases, death. These are just a few of the myriad of potential problems that all the behaviors of an eating disorder can cause. Some of these problems are reversible (depending on when the eating disorder is eliminated); some are not.

With compulsive overeating, there is the same cycle of dieting and binging present in the bulimic, except without the purging. Logically, compulsive overeaters are generally overweight, some morbidly so.

Although there may be some individual differences among people with eating disorders, the basics tend to be the same; namely, low self-esteem, body-image distortion, self-destructive behaviors, lack of control of food, and difficulty with extremely negative emotions. People with eating disorders are unhappy, despite how they may try to appear to others. These individuals feel out of control and are desperately trying to control their lives.

There are two main causes of eating disorders. The first is psychological. A perfectionistic personality underlying low self-esteem is the emotional root of the eating disorder. There has never been a case of an eating disorder in a person with a strong sense and liking of herself, who takes things in life in a relaxed manner and doesn't worry what others think about her. This type of person would never pursue something that clearly was making her unhappy and making her life get out of control. This is why one of the most essential goals of therapy for an eating disorder is to achieve total self-acceptance.

The second main cause of an eating disorder is a pattern of extreme dieting. As you've learned, dieting creates a state in the body of psychological and physiological deprivation. These in turn drive the person to eat by making her obsessed with food and resulting in loss of control with eating. Purging only serves to create a higher degree of deprivation. Starvation in other circumstances besides an eating disorder is known to produce symptoms of preoccupation with food (even dreaming about food). It also, to no surprise, causes malnutrition. When the brain is malnourished, it can't think straight, making it more difficult for the eating-disordered person to think logically and to problem-solve.

It's beyond the scope of this book to go into more detail about eating disorders, but, if any of this information feels familiar, it is suggested that you consult an expert in the field and find out if this is a problem that should be addressed. If an eating disorder does exist, continuing to solve weight issues without doing something about eliminating the eating disorder is going to result in another failure. In fact, most people with eating disorders have a long history of trying to control their problem with many methods, usually by more dieting and exercise, only to be disillusioned yet another time. Weight and food will always be issues in the life of the eating-disordered until the disorder is let go of forever.

And here we have the good news. It is very possible to get rid of an eating disorder entirely. By this, I mean that the eating-disordered person can again become a normal eating person whose life is not centered around food and weight, eats whenever she wants without concern or anxiety, uses healthy ways to stay fit and lean, and has total self-acceptance. However, in order to achieve this, the person has to: 1) realize that she has a serious problem and that this problem is not normal; 2) have a strong desire to be free of the eating disorder to the extent that she is willing to do anything that is not self-destructive to eliminate it; 3) seek professional and expert help for the problem; 4) realize that getting rid of the eating disorder is her responsibility and not the job of someone else; 5) be patient and accept the fact that a cure will be a gradual process with ups and downs; and 6) let go of all perfectionistic rules, not only about food, but about herself and her life.

The most effective treatments for eating disorders today include a cognitive/behavioral approach to psychotherapy, which helps the individual become aware of her dysfunctional thinking — the thinking that is keeping her stuck in a cyclical world of excessive control and loss of control of food and weight. It teaches the individual to dispute her dysfunctional thinking and to permanently replace it with thinking that is logical and results in feelings of natural control, relaxation, and contentment. There are many other therapy approaches that are also helpful, but without changing her thinking, the person with an eating disorder will remain at a disadvantage and cannot become her own therapist in life very easily.

A responsible and successful treatment program for someone with an eating disorder should also include training and knowledge about dieting, nutrition, and exercise. Without the proper nutrition, the body's demands to be fed adequately will make it harder for the person to do the other things required to eliminate the eating disorder. It's also necessary because the individual needs help in relearning to eat normally again — something that she knew naturally in the past. By learning about healthy eating and exercise, the eating-disordered person gains tools to be able to manage her weight in a positive, healthy, and successful way in the future, without compromising her life anymore.

The person with an eating disorder secretly desires to be free of it, to be someone who doesn't have to worry about what she eats or her weight anymore. She can be envious of others who she sees as being able to eat what they want peacefully without the imprisonment. It is definitely not fun to have an eating disorder. It's much harder than can be imagined by someone that's never been there. An eating disorder comes at a great cost to the individual that suffers from it, her loved ones and friends, and society. For all these reasons it is absolutely imperative that everyone involved understand the importance of getting treatment for the problem.

Here are some steps to take in finding help for an eating disorder:

- Read everything you can get your hands on about the problem.

- Look for a therapist who specializes in eating disorders. This person's caseload should be 90% cases or more of eating disorders.

- The therapy should be primarily individual therapy, rather than group therapy, as eating disorders require very intensive attention from the therapist.

- Steer away from any therapy that suggests that a cure can be achieved in a short period of time. One doesn't develop the eating disorder in a few days or weeks; a cure will not happen that quickly, either. Typically, one can expect to work in intensive therapy for at least a year.

- Also steer away from any therapy that suggests that you cannot be completely cured of an eating disorder, but, rather, you will have to be recovering for the rest of your life. There are many people walking around happily that used to have eating disorders and don't suffer from them to any extent anymore. A complete cure is available to you. Why settle for less?

- Interview more than one therapist before making a commitment. Ask many questions. Ask about the therapist's educational and ex-periential qualifications. The best therapists tend to have doctorates (either Ph.D., Psy.D., or M.D.), are licensed in their field, and are known in the community and outside of it as someone who is suc-cessful with treating eating disorders.

- You must like your therapist. He or she must be someone that makes you feel comfortable, listens, and talks to you in a kind yet direct manner. She or he will explain things thoroughly and will be patient. A good therapist will also be open to questions and invite questions from you.

- Don't look for the therapist to do all the work. Most of the work needs to come from you; if not, you will become dependent on that therapist and, what would you do when the therapy is over? Remember, the goal is to be your own therapist, to not need the therapist anymore so you can go about your life successfully on your own.

- Put your recovery first. If you don't, it won't happen.

- Be honest at all times with your therapist. She or he can't read your mind (although the good ones sometimes seem like they can). If you're not honest, you're the only one that's going to pay for it.

I realize that the tone of this chapter has been very different from that of the rest of this book. It was meant to be that way. While in earlier chapters we've focused on playfulness, letting go, getting rid of rules, and lightening up, the tone of this chapter has been very serious and almost ominous. An eating disorder isn't a light thing. It is not "nothing to worry about." It is a life and death issue. There are too many people out there silently suffering in the hell of an eating disorder that need help and deserve a happy life free of the bondage. These are the reasons for the tone of this chapter.

However, I hope the message is clear that it is absolutely unnecessary to continue to suffer with an eating disorder. It can be eliminated completely, and a person can be fit and lean, as well as be able to have a relationship with food, that's enjoyable and naturally controlled. Everyone deserves that — it's nature's way.

This book can be helpful to people with eating disorders by giving them accurate information, helping them to see what natural control of food is, and providing methods that can be used during and after therapy to help achieve complete recovery.

Chapter 21 Tidbits

- An eating disorder isn't something to be taken lightly. It can destroy your health, happiness, and social life. It can also cost you your life.

- Having an eating disorder will also keep you from having the best of all worlds — having natural control over food and being fit and lean.

- An eating disorder is a curable disorder. It's possible to be 100 percent free of it for the rest of your life.

- Recovering from an eating disorder requires patience and hard work, but it's well worth it because once you've recovered, you're done; whereas having an eating disorder is a never-ending cycle filled with misery and pain.

- A competent, likeable, and compassionate therapist makes the journey of recovery the easiest and most rewarding journey possible. It's always easier to have a knowledgeable guide when you're traveling somewhere you've never been before.

My "Mind Over Fat Matters" Notes

What I want to remember:

What I want to do:

How this will enrich my life:

Chapter 22

Conclusion:

The Power of the Mind

As you've seen, the brain can be a powerful ally or a stubborn enemy in your efforts to make changes with your weight. Most dieters' approaches to losing weight put the brain in a resistance mode, making it extremely difficult to follow their good intentions to eat well, exercise, and do other things that are supposed to result in weight loss.

You've also learned that when you unconsciously put yourself at a disadvantage against your brain, it would be wrong to blame yourself for your lack of success. It's a simple matter of not having enough information and not knowing the right things to do. When these truths are known, it is a freeing experience. You are no longer to blame for going through endless cycles of losing and gaining weight, from feeling like a quitter yet another time, or from feeling weak-willed. You now know that your brain will react with resistance to any negative, depriving, and judging approaches you try to use; therefore, you'll steer away from such methods.

You've learned that your thinking is central to your success with your weight. Rules are thoughts that demand perfection, which is impossible. Since rules are impossible to follow perfectly, it stands to reason that you'll be breaking them often and, based on your rules, this would mean that you've failed. Only thinking that is free of rules and filled, instead, with positive goals and incentives, playful images, and encouragement, will lead to success and allow you the freedom to learn through mistakes.

Your priorities in life determine your level of happiness and satisfaction with life. Priorities that don't include your inner peace, health, simple pleasures, and other such things will quickly bring you to an imbalance that will be hard to ignore. An eating disorder is an example of such an imbalance in life due to the wrong priorities.

Being as fit and lean as is reasonably possible is important in life. It helps you to enjoy more of the many wonderful things that life has to offer, including, but not of the greatest importance, being more attractive. Health gives you energy, allows you to do more things without as many obstacles from physical illness, and gives you more longevity. Health feels good, which helps in the happiness area. The reverse is also true; happiness helps you to gain and keep health. Health allows you to be more childlike, to play more with life.

Nutrition is a tool for gaining more health, for getting more enjoyment from the act of eating, and for preventing abnormal cravings that can lead to cycles of compulsive eating. Nutrition improves your appearance by giving you shinier hair, healthier skin, better muscle tone, brighter eyes, prettier smiles, and stronger bones for better posture. Yes, food is good — it is something to look forward to, not be afraid of, and it is what provides nutrition.

This book's attempt has been to give a fresh new perspective on the whole issue of weight management. It has also attempted to give insight into the reasons why so many people have trouble following well-known effective methods for weight control, such as a healthy food program and regular physical activity. In addition, it has argued that weight management can be a relatively simple and enjoyable process, not the drudgery that so many people have experienced over and over again. Weight control has been put within the realm of life in general; and the importance of making choices about weight management that will keep your life in balance has been demonstrated.

Finally, this book has provided step-by-step instructions on how to achieve success with weight in your life while maintaining this all-important balance. The hope is that this book will have challenged you, the reader, to make a commitment to solve any weight management problems, once-and for-all, by having the determination and courage to apply what works even if it's different from what others do or say. May you have a healthy, happy, and lean life, and may you always make choices based on what makes sense within the greater scheme of things. Remember the child in you.

My "Mind Over Fat Matters" Notes

What I want to remember:

What I want to do:

How this will enrich my life:

Dr. Lavinia Rodriguez is a bilingual, clinical psychologist and an expert in eating disorders and weight management. She has extensive public speaking experience in the areas of weight, eating and exercise, as well as many other mental health issues, including relationships, anxiety, dysfunctional thinking, and self-esteem. She has authored articles in Active Living (September/October 1999) and Working Together, the National Association of Anorexia Nervosa and Associated Disorders (ANAD) newsletter, and has been quoted as an expert on eating disorders in Weight Watchers Magazine (July 1991).

"The highlight of my professional life as a psychologist has been to serve as a guide to countless people of all ages who have struggled with weight and eating issues. Typically, these people have experienced repeated failures despite their best intentions. To see the joy in their faces and the improvement in the quality of their lives after working with someone who could show them how to finally make it work has added tremendously to my life as a psychologist and a person."

The author has lived in the Tampa Bay Area since 1971. "I am married to a true partner in life and we both enjoy our lives in an 'Old Florida' setting surrounded by water, cypress and colorful gardens—the perfect home for our three cats: Louise, Domino and Tupelo Honey."

Printed in the United States
149255LV00003B/2/P